The Guru Method

WorkBook – Sections I and II

This book is copyright. Apart from any fair dealing for the purposes of private study, research, criticism or review as permitted under the Copyright Act, no part of this publication may be reproduced, stored in a retrieval system, or transmitted in any form or by any means, electronic, mechanical, photocopying, recording or otherwise without prior written permission.

For information contact:

GSMS Education Pty Ltd
P.O Box 3848
Marsfield NSW
2122
Australia

Practice Questions – Section I & II

Welcome to WorkBook #1 - Section I and II Practice Questions. The aim of this workbook is to develop your reading, writing and comprehension skills to a level required for you to excel at Section I & II in the GAMSAT.

Table of Contents

PRACTICE QUESTIONS – SECTION I & II 3

LITERATURE 7
  UNIT 1 - CHARLES DICKENS "HARD TIMES" 7
  UNIT 2 - ERKSINE CALDWELL "GOD'S LITTLE ACRE" 10
  UNIT 3 - JANE AUSTEN "MANSFIELD PARK" 13
  UNIT 4 - MORRIS WEST "THE DEVIL'S ADVOCATE" 17
  UNIT 5 - JOHN STEINBECK "OF MICE AND MEN" 19
  UNIT 6 - WILLIAM BOOTH "IN DARKEST ENGLAND AND THE WAY OUT" 22

PHILOSOPHY 25
  UNIT 7 - MACHIAVELLI "THE PRINCE" 25
  UNIT 8 - JEAN-JACQUES ROUSSEAU "THE SOCIAL CONTRACT" 27
  UNIT 9 - HENRY DAVID THOREAU "CIVIL DISOBEDIENCE" 31
  UNIT 10 - FRANCIS BACON "NOVUM ORGANUM" 33
  UNIT 11 - QUOTATIONS 35

CARTOONS 37
  UNIT 12 - BUSH AND PUTIN'S DEMOCRACY DRIVING 37
  UNIT 13 - IVF 38
  UNIT 14 - LONG-TERM US ENERGY POLICY 39
  UNIT 15 - ANOTHER FOOD PYRAMID 40
  UNIT 16 - WAR ON TERROR 41
  UNIT 17 - MANAGEMENT 43
  UNIT 18 - GOVERNMENT MINISTER 45
  UNIT 19 - BUSINESS 47
  UNIT 20 - SAME SEX 48
  UNIT 21 - BOYFRIEND 50
  UNIT 22 - BEACH 51
  UNIT 23 - CONVERSATION 53
  UNIT 24 - PETROL 55
  UNIT 25 - RITUAL 57

POETRY 59
  UNIT 26 - GWENDOLYN BROOKS "KITCHENETTE BUILDING" 59
  UNIT 27 - LOUIS MACNIECE "SONG" 61
  UNIT 28 - HUMBERT WOLFE "THE GREY SQUIRREL" 63
  UNIT 29 - LINDA PASTAN "ETHICS" 65
  UNIT 30 - DAME MARY GILMORE "EVE-SONG" 67
  UNIT 31 - PERCY BYSSHE SHELLEY "OZYMANDIAS" 70
  UNIT 32 - G. ESSEX EVANS "THE WOMAN ON THE WEST" 72
  UNIT 33 - JOHN KEATS "THE HUMAN SEASONS" 75

SOCIOLOGY 77
  UNIT 34 - DANIEL BELL "MODERNISN, POSTMODERNISM
            AND THE DECLINE OF MORAL ORDER" 77

AUSTRALIAN 81
  UNIT 35 - CHLOE HOOPER "A CHILD'S BOOK OF TRUE CRIME" 81
  UNIT 36 - PAUL KELLY "THE CHANGES, THE CHALLENGES,
            THE CHOICES FOR AUSTRALIA" 84
  UNIT 37 - ROBERT HUGHES "THE FATAL SHORE" 87
  UNIT 38 - STEPHEN J. PYNE "BURNING BUSH" 89
  UNIT 39 - THOMAS KENEALLY "OUTBACK" 91
  UNIT 40 - DAVID MALOUF "CLOSER" 93
  UNIT 41 - EVE D. FESI 96

MODERN PROSE 98
  UNIT 42 - D.J. WALDIE "HOLY LAND: A SUBURBAN MEMOIR" 98
  UNIT 43 - ITALO CALVINO "SIX MEMOS FOR THE NEXT MILLENNIUM" 100
  UNIT 44 - KEITH BASSO "WISDOM SITS IN PLACES" 102
  UNIT 45 - "SOLDIERS AGAINST CRIME, OR
            POLICE IN A COMMUNITY?" 104
  UNIT 46 - TIM WINTON "DIRT MUSIC" 106
  UNIT 47 - SAMUEL ALEXANDER "SPACE, TIME AND DEITY, VOL. 1" 108
  UNIT 48 - "GOVERNMENT NOT RATTLED BY FUEL POLICY ATTACK" 111

CONCEPTUAL THINKING 114
UNIT 49 - SIGNAL FLARES 114
UNIT 50 - DRUG TESTING 117
UNIT 51 - DOG COAT COLOUR 120
UNIT 52 - MAP READING 123
UNIT 53 - MEMORY ACCESS 127
UNIT 54 - PLANT GROWTH 130
UNIT 55 - VOTING SYSTEMS 133

SECTION II ESSAY TOPICS 137
CREATIVITY 137
DEFEAT 138
IMMORTALITY 139
OPPORTUNITY 140
PATRIOTISM 141
MATURITY 142
MONEY 143
RISK 144
WAR 145
TEMPTATION 146

WORKED SOLUTIONS 147

Literature

UNIT 1 - Charles Dickens "Hard Times"

Excerpt from Charles Dickens *"Hard Times"*

It was a town of red brick, or of brick that would have been red if the smoke and ashes had allowed it; but as matters stood it was a town of unnatural red and black, like the painted face of a savage. It was a town of machinery and tall chimneys, out of which interminable serpents of smoke trailed themselves for ever and ever, and never got uncoiled. It had a black canal in it, and a river that ran purple with ill-smelling dye, and vast piles of building full of windows where there was a rattling and a trembling all day long, and where the piston of the steam engine worked monotonously up and down, like the head of an elephant in a state of melancholy madness. It contained several large streets all very like one another, and many small streets still more like one another, inhabited by people equally like one another, who all went in and out at the same hours, with the same sound upon the same pavements, to do the same work, and to whom every day was the same as yesterday and tomorrow, and every year the counterpart of the last and the next.

These attributes of Coketown were in the main inseparable from the work by which it was sustained. Against them were to be set off comforts of life which found their way all over the world, and elegancies of life which made, we will not ask how much of the fine lady, who could scarcely bear to hear the place mentioned. The rest of its features were voluntary, and they were these.

You saw nothing in Coketown but what was severely workful. If the members of a religious persuasion built a chapel there—as the members of eighteen religious persuasions had done—they made it a pious warehouse of red brick, with sometimes (but this only in highly ornamented examples) a bell in a birdcage on the top of it. The solitary exception was the New Church, a stuccoed edifice with a square steeple over the door, terminating in four short pinnacles like

florid wooden legs. All the public inscriptions in the town were
painted alike, in severe characters of black and white. The jail might
have been the infirmary, the infirmary might have been the jail, the
town-hall might have been either, or both, or anything else, for
anything that appeared to the contrary in the graces of their
construction. Fact, fact, fact, everywhere in the material aspect of
the town; fact, fact, fact, everywhere in the immaterial. The
M'Choakumchild school was all fact, and the school of design was all
fact, and the relations between master and man were all fact, and
everything was fact between the lying-in hospital and the cemetery,
and what you couldn't state in figures, or show to be purchasable in
the cheapest market and saleable in the dearest, was not, and never
should be, world without end. Amen.

1. The imagery used by Dickens in this passage, such as 'red bricks', 'black canal', 'serpents of smoke' is to depict Coketown as

    A an unnatural place
    B an industrial hell
    C an uninhabitable place
    D a soulless place

2. It may be inferred that Dickens' portrayal of Coketown is intended

    A to show a town suffering from malaise
    B to be a severe critique of the spillover cost of a market economy
    C as a criticism of irresponsible proprietorship
    D to decry consumerism

3. "All the public inscriptions in the town were painted alike, in black and white."
   The two colours, "black and white" imply that

    A there are only two values to be considered – right and wrong.
    B there is no artistic talent in the town
    C no one can see any shades in moral issues.
    D everything is regulated to be functional and basic.

Literature — 9

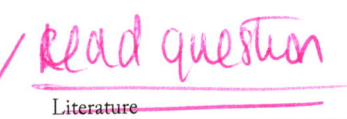

Read question

4 Which value does (not) exist in Coketown as portrayed by Dickens?

    A Utility
    B Imagination
    (C) Materialism
    D Class consciousness ✗

it is true that everything has to be facts, facts, facts and that imagination cannot exist

5 In this passage, Dickens is in reality

    (A) implicitly presenting a case for the people left without legal or popular counsel.
    B ascribing blame on entrepreneurs.
    C condemning a sterile religion.
    D supporting the theory that all things must be useful.

basically he talks about the dreadful routine

UNIT 2 - Erksine Caldwell "God's Little Acre"

Excerpt from Erksine Caldwell's *God's Little Acre*. It tells the story of industrial situation during the depression.

Will had turned and was pointing out the window towards the darkened cotton mill. There was no light in the huge building, but arc lights under the trees threw a thin coating of yellow glow over the ivy covered walls.
"When's the mill going to start up again? Pluto asked.
"Never," Will said disgustedly. "Never. Unless we start it ourselves."
"What's the matter? Why won't it run?"
Will leaned forward in his chair.
"We're going in there some day ourselves and turn the power on," he said slowly. "If the company doesn't start up soon, that's what we're going to do. They cut the pay down to a dollar-ten eighteen months ago, and when we raised hell about it, they shut off the power and drove us out. But they still charge rent for these God damn privies we have to live in. You know why we're going to run it ourselves now, don't you?"
"But some of the other mills in the Valley are running," Pluto said. "We passed five or six lighted mills when we drove over from Augusta tonight. Maybe they'll start this one again soon."
"Like so much hell they will, at a dollar-ten. They are running the pother mills because they starved the loomweavers into going back to work. That was before the Red Cross started passing out sacks of flour. They had to go back to work and take a dollar-ten, or starve. But, by God, we don't have to do it in Scottsville. As long as we can get a sack of flour once in a while we can hold out. And the State is giving out yeast now. Mix a cake of yeast in a glass of water and drink it, and you feel pretty good for a while. They started giving out yeast because everybody in the Valley has got pellagra these days from too much starving. The mill can't get us back until they shorten the hours, or cut out the stretchout, or go back to the old pay. I'll be damned if I work nine hours a day for a dollar-ten, when those rich sons-of-bitches who own the mill ride up and down the Valley in five thousand dollar automobiles.
Will had got warmed to the subject, and once started, he could not stop. He told Pluto something of their plans for taking over the mill from the owners and running it themselves. The mill workers in Scottsville had been out of work for a year and a half already, he said, and they were becoming desperate for food and clothing. During that length of time the workers had reached an understanding among

themselves that bound every man, woman, and child in the company town to a stand not to give in to the mill. The mill had tried to evict them from their homes for nonpayment of rent, but the local had got an injunction from a judge in Aiken that restrained the mill from turning the workers out of the company houses. With that, Will said, they were prepared to stand for their demands just as long as the mill stood in Scottsville.

6 Will, the character in the passage, is talking about

I exploitation by the owners of capital.
II a strike.
III a union disaster.
IV an unfair dismissal problem..

Which of the following is true?

    A Statement I only.
    B Statements I, II and IV.
    C Statement III only.
    D Statement II only.

7 Pluto, the other character in the passage is set up as a simpleton. His role is to help create

    A tension in the narrative.
    B an audience for Will's anger.
    C a foil to Will.
    D a dialogue for narrative flow.

8 Which of the following is not included in "symbolic violence" by the mill owners against the workers?

    A Reducing the workers' pay.
    B Giving yeast to mix a drink.
    C Starvation.
    D Raising rents of the "God damn privies".

9 Which of the following is a condition for not withholding labour?

   A Shortening the hours.
   B Abolishing the time extension.
   C Recourse to previous pay.
   D Increasing workers' pay.

10 The heart of this story lies in the concept of

   A economic competition
   B economic inequality
   C the cash nexus.
   D control of capital.

UNIT 3 - Jane Austen "Mansfield Park"

Passage from Jane Austen's *Mansfield Park*

About 30 years ago, Miss Maria Ward of Huntingdon, with only seven thousand pounds, had the good luck to captivate Sir Thomas Bertram, of Mansfield Park, in the county of Northampton, and to be thereby raised the rank of a baronet's lady, with all the comforts and consequences of a handsome house and large income. All Huntingdon exclaimed on the greatness of the match and her uncle, the lawyer, himself, allowed her to be at least three thousand pounds short of any equitable claim to it. She had two sisters to be benefited by her elevation; and such of their acquaintance as thought Miss Ward and Miss Frances quite as handsome as Miss Maria, did not scruple to predict their marrying with almost equal advantage. But there certainly are not so many men of large fortune in the world, as there are pretty women to deserve them. Miss Ward, at the end of hall a dozen years, found herself obliged to be attached to the Rev. Mr. Norris, a friend of her brother-in-law, with scarcely any private fortune, and Miss Frances fared yet worse. Miss. Ward's match, indeed, when it came to the point, was not contemptible. Sir Thomas being happily able to give his friend an income in the living of Mansfield, and Mr. and Mrs. Norris began their career of conjugal felicity with very little less than a thousand a year. But Miss Frances married, in the common phrase, to disoblige her family, and by fixing on a Lieutenant of Marines, without education, fortune, or connections, did it very well.

11 This passage, with its beginning "About thirty years ago ...." has a tone of

   A conversation
   B gossip
   C nostalgia
   D gravity

Practice Questions - Section I and II

12 The words "with only seven thousand pounds", " had the good luck", "comforts and consequences" reflect an acute sense of a society's awareness of the fundamental ingredient of

   A social status
   B honour
   C privilege
   D class

13 "All Huntingdon exclaimed on the greatness of the match." The author is communicating to the reader the social role of

   A intrusiveness
   B gossip
   C approval
   D envy

14 In the context of the passage, which of the following is not considered an essential determinant for marriage?

   A Social status of the male
   B Class
   C Income
   D Love

15 Though some of the sisters' acquaintances did not scruple to predict that they would marry 'with nearly equal advantage, Miss Ward, at the end of half a dozen years, found herself obliged to be attached to the Rev. Mr. Norris, a friend of her brother-in-law, with scarcely any private fortune…'. This expresses

A an ironic situation
B the disaster of Miss Ward's life
C the necessity of obeying social convention
D the hand of fate

16 'But Miss Frances married, in the common phrase, to disoblige her family, and by fixing on a lieutenant of marines, without education, fortune, or connections, did it very thoroughly'. This underlined phrase means

A she thoroughly put an end to all relationship with her family.
B she brought disgrace to her family.
C her family were glad to get rid of her.
D she did not care at all whom she married.

17 From the passage, which description is not true of Sir Thomas Bertram's character?

A He is a conceited man.
B He is a man of principle.
C He is a person who is aware of family ties.
D He has the capacity to use his connections for good.

18 In recounting the marriages of the three sisters, Jane Austen reveals to the reader

    A the pitfalls of marriage.
    B the predetermined countless pressures that accompany the institution of marriage.
    C the necessity to marry soon and to advantage.
    D the stigmatized marriage.

(B) as it covers all A, C + D

UNIT 4 - Morris West "The Devil's Advocate"

This is the opening of Morris West's novel 'The Devil's Advocate'.

It was his profession to prepare other men for death; it shocked him to be so unready for his own. He was a reasonable man and reason told him that a man's death sentence is written on his palm the day he is born; he was a cold man, little troubled by passion, irked not at all by discipline, yet his first impulse had been a wild clinging to the illusion of immortality.

It was part of the decency of Death that he should come unheralded with face covered and hands concealed, at the hour when he was least expected. He should come slowly, softly, like his brother sleep—or swiftly and violently like the consummation of the act of love, so that the moment of surrender would be a stillness and satiety instead of a wrenching separation of spirit and flesh.

The decency of Death. It was the thing men hoped for vaguely, prayed for if they were disposed to pray regretted bitterly when they knew it would be denied them. Blaise Meredith was regretting it now, as he sat in the thin spring sunshine, watching the slow processional swans on the Serpentine, the courting couples on the grass, the leashed poodles trotting fastidiously along the paths at the flirting skirts of their owners.

19 The author stimulates our interest in the opening of this novel by

   A making us wonder who this character, 'whose profession is to prepare other men for death' is.
   B by using shock tactics through emotive words such as 'death' and 'shock'.
   C by using prediction.
   D all of the above.

20 The introduction says, 'It was his profession to prepare other men for death; it shocked him to be so unready for his own.' The most likely reason for this is:

   A He had never pondered upon his own demise.
   B A reversal of situation.
   C An unexpected revelation.
   D Human avoidance of the truth.

Practice Questions - Section I and II

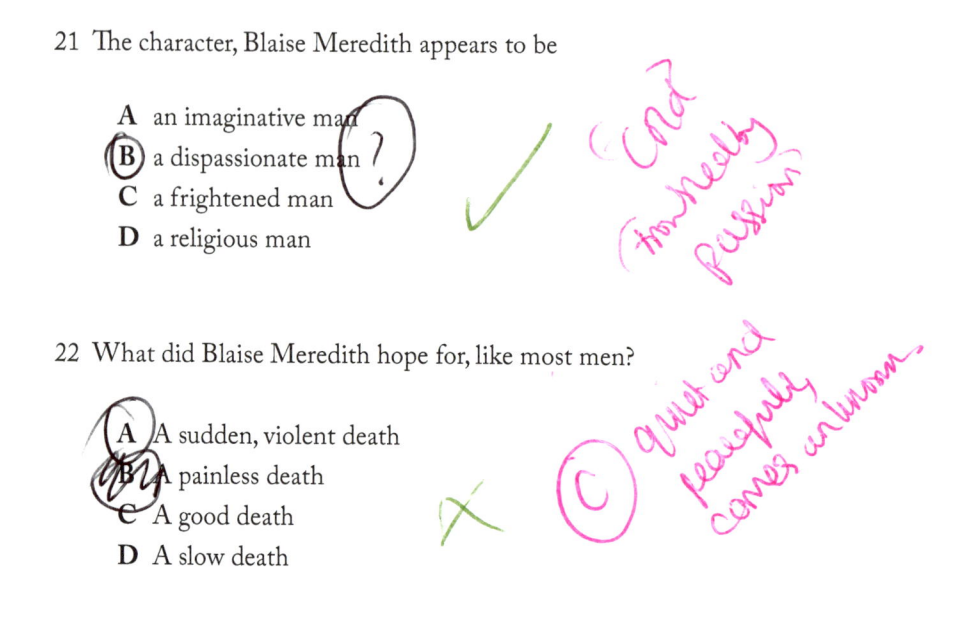

21 The character, Blaise Meredith appears to be

    A an imaginative man
    B a dispassionate man
    C a frightened man
    D a religious man

22 What did Blaise Meredith hope for, like most men?

    A A sudden, violent death
    B A painless death
    C A good death
    D A slow death

23 The atmosphere created by this piece of writing is one of

    A peace and resignation
    B soberness and regret
    C bitterness
    D quiet contemplation

24 The vividness of the description of the park is to

    A depict the author's skill at description.
    B reveal the character's cold contemplation in the light of day.
    C create an atmosphere of peace.
    D offer a stark contrast between the dark thoughts of the character and the liveliness of a bright, beautiful day.

UNIT 5 - John Steinbeck "Of Mice and Men"

This passage is an excerpt from *Of Mice and Men* by John Steinbeck.

The ranch hands have all gone to town, leaving Crooks (the African – American), Candy, (an old man) and Lennie (who is intellectually challenged) behind.

Candy stood in the doorway scratching his bald wrist and looking blindly into the lighted room. He made no attempt to enter. 'Tell ya what, Lennie. I been figuring out about them rabbits.'
Crooks said irritably: 'You can come in if you want.'
Candy seemed embarrassed. 'I do' know. 'Course, if ya want me to.'
'Come on in. If ever'body's comin' in, you might just as well.' It was difficult for Crooks to conceal his pleasure with anger.
Candy came in, but he was still embarrassed. 'You got a nice cosy little place in here,' he said to Crooks. 'Must be nice to have a room all to yourself this way.'
'Sure,' said Crooks. 'And a manure pile under the window. Sure it's swell.'
Lennie broke in: 'You said about them rabbits.'
Candy leaned against the wall beside the broken collar while he scratched the wrist stump. 'I been here a long time,' he said. 'An' Crooks been here a long time. This's the first time I ever been in his room.'
Crooks said darkly: 'Guys don't come into a coloured man's room very much. Nobody been here but Slim. Slim an' the boss.'
Candy quickly changed the subject. 'Slim's as good a skinner as I ever seen.'
Lennie leaned toward the old swamper. 'About them rabbits,' he insisted.
Candy smiled. 'I got figured out. We can make some money on them rabbits if we go about it right.'
'But I get to tend 'em,' Lennie broke in. 'George says I get to tend 'em. He promised.'
Crooks interrupted brutally. 'You guys is just kiddin' yourself. You'll talk about it a hell of a lot, but you won't get no land. You'll be a swamper here till they take you out in a box. Hell, I seen too many guys. Lennie here'll quit an' be on the road in two, three weeks. Seems like ever' guy got land in his head.'
Candy rubbed his cheek angrily. 'You God damn right we're gonna do it. George says we are. We got the money right now.'
'Yeah?' said Crooks. 'An' where's George now? In town in a whore-house. That's where your money's goin'. Jesus, I seen it happen too many times. I seen too many guys with land in their head. They never get none under their hand.'
Candy cried: 'Sure they all want it. Everybody wants a little bit of land, not

much. Jus' som'thin' that was his. Som'thin' he could live on and there couldn't nobody throw him off of it. I never had none. I planted crops for damn near ever'body in this state, but they wasn't my crops, and when I harvested 'em, it wasn't none of my harvest. But we gonna do it now, and don't you make no mistake about that. George ain't got the money in town. That money's in the bank. Me an' Lennie an' George. We gonna have a room to ourselves. We're gonna have a dog an' rabbits an' chickens. We're gonna have green corn an' maybe a cow or a goat.' He stopped, overwhelmed with his picture.
Crooks asked: 'You say you got the money?'
'Damn right. We got most of it. Just a little bit more to get.
Have it all in one month. George got the land all picked out, too.'
Crooks reached around and explored his spine with his hand. 'I never seen a guy really do it,' he said. 'I seen guys nearly crazy with loneliness for land, but ever' time a whorehouse or a blackjack game took what it takes.' He hesitated.'... If you ... guys would want a hand to work for nothing—just his keep, why I'd come an' lend a hand. I ain't so crippled I can't work like a son-of-a-bitch if I want to.'

25 Crooks' hostility at the 'home invasion' is a cover for his

   A loneliness
   B fear
   C embarrassment
   D desire to socialise

26 When Crooks scornfully says: 'Seems like ever' guy got land in his head', he addresses a focal issue of the author. This issue is:

   A Men like to dream.
   B One should rise above survival from one day to the next
   C There is an unfailing aspiration even in the lowliest of men.
   D Many men are merely drifters.

Literature

27 When Candy cried: 'Sure they all want it. Everybody wants a little bit of land, not much. Jus' som'thin' that was his. Som'thin' he could live on and there couldn't nobody throw him off of it.' He voices the human need for

    A security
    B ownership
    C commitment
    D selfhood

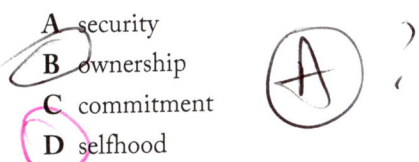

28 Crooks capitulate and indicates that he wants to join Candy and Lennie because

    A he too has ambition.
    B of an innate need to feel connected.
    C he does not wish to be sidelined.
    D he hates the ranch.

29 Steinbeck's attitude to these single, homeless men is one of

    A contempt
    B condescension
    C compassion and understanding
    D sentimentality

UNIT 6 - William Booth "In Darkest England and the Way Out"

William Booth (1829–1919) was a religious and social reformer who founded the Salvation Army. He drew the extended analogy for In Darkest England from a variety of Victorian narratives of exploration, especially Henry Stanley's best-selling account of his travels through Africa, Through the Dark Continent (1879). Booth hoped to solve the problem of urban poverty by developing work colonies in Great Britain and abroad.

Passage from William Booth: In Darkest England and the Way Out (1890)

Why "Darkest England"?

This summer the attention of the civilized world has been arrested by the story which Mr. Stanley has told of "Darkest Africa" and his journeys across the heart of the Lost Continent. In all that spirited narrative of heroic endeavor, nothing has so much impressed the imagination, as his description of the immense forest, which offered an almost impenetrable barrier to his advance. The intrepid explorer, in his own phrase, "marched, tore, ploughed, and cut his way for one hundred and sixty days through this inner womb of the true tropical forest."

The mind of man with difficulty endeavors to realize this immensity of wooded wilderness, covering a territory half as large again as the whole of France, where the rays of the sun never penetrate, where in the dark, dank air, filled with the steam of the heated morass, human beings dwarfed into pygmies and brutalized into cannibals lurk and live and die. Mr. Stanley vainly endeavors to ring home to us the full horror of that awful gloom.

It is a terrible picture, and one that has engraved itself deep on the heart of civilization. But while brooding over the awful presentation of life as it exists in the vast African forest, it seemed to me only too vivid a picture of many parts of our own land. As there is a darkest Africa is there not also a darkest England? Civilization, which can breed its own barbarians, does it not also breed its own pygmies? May we not find a parallel at our own doors, and discover within a stone's throw of our cathedrals and palaces similar horrors to those which Stanley has found existing in the great Equatorial forest?

The more the mind dwells upon the subject, the closer the analogy appears. The ivory raiders who brutally traffic in the unfortunate denizens of the forest glades, what are they but the publicans who flourish on the weakness of our poor? The two tribes of savages, the human baboon and the handsome dwarf, who will not speak lest it impede him in his task, may be accepted as the two varieties who are continually present with us — the vicious, lazy lout, and the toiling slave. They, too, have lost all faith of life being other than it is and has been. As in Africa, it is all trees, trees, trees with no other world conceivable; so is it here — it is all vice and poverty and crime. To many the world is all slum, with the Workhouse as an intermediate purgatory before the grave. And just as Mr. Stanley's Zanzibaris lost faith, and could only be induced to plod on in brooding sullenness of dull despair, so the most of our social reformers, no matter how cheerily they may have started off, with forty pioneers swinging blithely their axes as they force their way into the wood, soon become depressed and despairing. Who can battle against the ten thousand million trees? Who can hope to make headway against the innumerable adverse conditions which doom the dweller in Darkest England to eternal and immutable misery?

30 The intention of the writer of this article intended to

    A criticize the 'civilized world'.
    B arouse public attention to social conditions of the time.
    C pour scorn on the indifference of the authorities
    D describe the exploitation of the poor.

31 To make this article effective, Booth uses the analogy of

    A the dark and immense forest
    B hell
    C the ivory raiders
    D the slum

32 According to the article, there is no way out for the majority of the urban poor because they are

    A victims of the publicans
    B lazy and vicious
    C existing in continual hopelessness
    D their numbers counteract the efforts of the reformers.

33 The tone of the article is one of

　　A intense anger and despair
　　B compassion and frustration
　　C a sense of failure
　　D a sense of powerlessness

34 This passage presents

　　A a comparison between England and Africa.
　　B an indictment of the social injustices of the day
　　C a description of the weak and exploited.
　　D the state of unconcern by those in 'cathedrals and palaces'.

Philosophy

UNIT 7 - Machiavelli "The Prince"

Passage from Machiavelli: *The Prince* first translated from Latin 1640.

One might well wonder how it was that Agathocles, and others like him, after countless treacheries and cruelties, could live securely in his own country and hold foreign enemies at bay, with never a conspiracy against him by his countrymen, in as much as many others, because of their cruel behaviour, have not been able to maintain their rule even in peaceful times, let alone in the uncertain times of war. I believe that here it is a question of cruelty used well or badly. We can say that cruelty is used well (if it is permissible to talk in this way of what is evil) when it is employed once for all, and one's safety depends on it and then it is not persisted in but as far as possible turned to the good of one's subjects. Cruelty badly used is that which although infrequent to start with/as time goes on, rather than disappearing, becomes more evident. Those who use the first method can, with divine and human assistance, find some means of consolidating their position, as did Agathocles; the others cannot possibly stay in power.
So it should be noted that when he seizes a state the new ruler ought to determine all the injuries that he will need to inflict. He should inflict them once for all and not have to renew them every day, and in that way he will be able to set men's minds at rest and win them over to him when he confers benefits. Whoever acts otherwise either through timidity or bad advice, is always forced to have the knife ready in his hand and he can never depend on his subjects because they, suffering fresh and continuous violence, can never feel secure with regard to him.

Violence should be inflicted once for all; people will then forget what it tastes like and so be less resentful. Benefits should be conferred gradually; and in that way they will taste better. Above all, a prince should live with his subjects in such a way that no development, either favourable or adverse, makes him vary of his conduct. When adversity brings the need for it, repression is too late; and the favours he may confer are profitless, because they are seen is being forced, and so they earn no thanks.

35 The cruel Agathocles was able to preserve his power, holding enemies at bay because he was

    A crafty
    B immoral
    C resourceful
    D pragmatic

36 Machiavelli argues that methods of government, though immoral, will be effective if applied

    A infrequently
    B consistently
    C intensely
    D frequently

37 Which of the following do not form part of Machiavelli's advice to the prince?

    A Use violence judiciously.
    B If seizing a state, sum up the injuries that has to be inflicted.
    C Confer rewards to consolidate your allies as soon as possible.
    D Enable your subjects to feel secure.

38 The main purpose of this passage is to

    A demonstrate raw political power.
    B promote effective procedures for maintaining a state
    C justify conquest.
    D illustrate that good government is equated to the character and skill of the individual leader.

UNIT 8 - Jean-Jacques Rousseau "The Social Contract"

This excerpt is from Jean-Jacques Rousseau's *"The Social Contract"*, written in 1743

I assume that men reach a point where the obstacles to their preservation in a state of nature prove greater than the strength that each man has to preserve himself in that state. Beyond this point, the primitive condition cannot endure, for then the human race will perish if it does not change its mode of existence. Since men cannot create new forces, but merely combine and control those which already exist, the only way in which they can preserve themselves is by uniting their separate powers in a combination strong enough to overcome any resistance, uniting them so that their powers are directed by a single motive and act in concert.

Such a sum of forces can be produced only by the union of separate men, but as each man's own strength and liberty are the chief instruments of his preservation, how can he merge his with others' without putting himself in peril and neglecting the care he owes to himself? This difficulty, which brings me back to my present subject, may be expressed in these words:

'How to find a form of association which will defend the person and goods of each member with the collective force of all, and under which each individual, while uniting himself with the others, obeys no one but himself, and remains as free as before.' This is the fundamental problem to which the social contract holds the solution. The articles of this contract are so precisely determined by the nature of the act, that the slightest modification must render them null and void; they are such that, though perhaps never formally stated, they are everywhere the same, everywhere tacitly admitted and recognized; and if ever the social pact is violated, every man regains his original rights and, recovering his natural freedom, loses that social freedom for which he exchanged it.

These articles of association, rightly understood, are reducible to a single one, namely the total alienation by each associate of himself and all his rights to the whole community. Thus, in the first place, as every individual gives himself absolutely, the conditions are the same for all, and precisely because they are the same for all, it is in no one's interest to make the conditions onerous for others.

Secondly, since the alienation is unconditional, the union is as perfect as it could be, and no individual associate has any longer any rights to claim; for if rights were left to individuals, in the absence of any higher authority to judge between them and the public, each individual, being his own judge in some causes, would soon demand to be his own judge in all; and in this way the state of nature would be kept in being, and the association inevitably become either tyrannical or void.

Finally, since each man gives himself to all, he gives himself to no one; and since there is no associate over whom he does not gain the same rights as others gain over him, each man recovers the equivalent of everything he loses, and in the bargain he acquires more power to preserve what he has.

If, then, we eliminate from the social pact everything that is not essential to it, we find it comes down to this: 'Each one of us puts into the community his person and all his powers under the supreme direction of the general will; and as a body, we incorporate every member as an indivisible part of the whole.

39 In the first paragraph, Rousseau's basic assumption is that man in a state of nature or pre-political condition

    A cannot sustain himself because of threats such as rising population.
    B will perish as his knowledge and strength become insufficient in the face of overwhelming dangers.
    C has little organizational skills to formulate laws which would safeguard his liberty.
    D has little imagination on how to form groups.

40 In paragraph 3 and 4, Rousseau poses the problem of how to establish

    A a society in which everyone must obey the legal structures
    B a social order based on freedom and equality founded on an implicit and mutual pact.
    C a cooperative community.
    D an association of individuals working together.

Philsophy

41 When Rousseau says that 'in the new state we remain as free as before', he is indicating

    A that individuals have the inherent capacity to resist oppression.
    B a body that is unencumbered by any institutions such as the police.
    C that everyone is now above the law.
    D that the new social contract will guarantee individual autonomy.

42 Which of the following would Rousseau's social contract not include?

    A Voluntary membership.
    B A mandate of specific behaviour that must be agreed upon on pain of losing his social freedom.
    C A basic agreement by all citizens regarding their rights and obligations
    D Laws and regulations infringing upon the basic contract, less it be rendered annulled.

43 By the term "total alienation" (paragraph 6, line 2), Rousseau means

    A an absolute transference of an individual and his rights to the state.
    B an illegitimate surrender of individual rights to the state.
    C an estrangement of the individual from the community.
    D state usurpation of individual rights and freedom.

44 In paragraph 7 which begins: "Finally, since each man gives himself to all…………." we can surmise that the social contract as such, is

    A a no-win situation
    B a win-lose situation
    C a zero-sum situation
    D a win-win situation

45 Rousseau's concept of the "general will" can be explained as

    A the embodiment of consensus in society, not the private will of its members.
    B the absolute abrogation of personal rights.
    C what will most benefit all.
    D the freedom of all

UNIT 9 - Henry David Thoreau "Civil Disobedience"

This is a passage from "Civil Disobedience" written by Henry David Thoreau in 1849. Thoreau refused to pay his poll tax to the government in order to make his disapproval of the Mexican War provoked by America, known. Since a portion of this money would go to the military budget for the war, Thoreau refused to contribute and he had to spend a night in jail. He was released because an unknown person paid the tax on his behalf.

> But to speak practically and as a citizen, unlike those who call themselves no-government men. I ask for, not at once no government, but at once a better government. Let every man make known what kind of government would command his respect, and that will be one step toward obtaining it. After all, the practical reason why, when the power is once in the hands of the people, a majority is permitted, and for a long period continue, is not because they are most likely to be right, nor because this seems fairest to the majority, but because they are physically the strongest. But a government in which the majority rule in all cases cannot be based on justice, even as far as men understand it. Can there not be a government in which majorities do not virtually decide what is right and wrong, but conscience? – in which majorities decide only those questions to which the rule of expediency is applicable? Must the citizen ever for a moment, or in the least degree, resign his conscience to the legislation? Why has every man a conscience, then? I think we should be men first, and subjects afterward. It is not desirable to cultivate a respect for the law so much as for the right.

46 Thoreau writes : "To speak practically...". By this he means

    A his concerns must have a chance of fulfillment.
    B he is not being merely idealistic.
    C he is not asking his listeners to follow a dream.
    D he has thought about his concerns thoroughly.

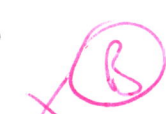

47 To Thoreau, "better government" is one

    A based on the rule of the majority.
    B based on the rule of law.
    C based on personal conscience.
    D based on the fewest number of laws.

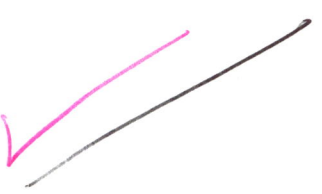

48 "A government in which the majority rules in all cases cannot be based on justice." This is because

   A such a government is based on "might is right".
   B right and wrong is not a question of the wielders of power but of conscience.
   C any law, invasive and pervasive, can be passed by the majority.
   D those who disagree are called anti-government.

49 "I think we should be men first, and subjects afterwards." This sentence implies that

   A men should have the courage of their convictions.
   B it is desirable to cultivate a respect for government.
   C the writer is encouraging civil disobedience in all cases of injustice.
   D there is a need to negotiate with the majority sometimes.

50 What is this passage not saying?

   A A government ought to act only on the practical aspects of ruling.
   B A tyranny of the majority cannot be tolerated.
   C Citizens are under no obligation to obey any unjust law.
   D Citizens should have a healthy respect for the law.

UNIT 10 - Francis Bacon "Novum Organum"

The following is an extract from 'Novum Organum' written by Francis Bacon.

Those who have taken upon them to lay down the law of nature as a thing already searched out and understood, whether they have spoken in simple assurance or professional affectation, have therein done philosophy and the sciences great injury. For as they have been successful in inducing belief, so they have been effective in quenching and stopping inquiry; and have done more harm by spoiling and putting an end to other men's efforts than good by their own.

Those on the other hand who have taken a contrary course, and asserted that absolutely nothing can be known – whether it were from hatred of the ancient sophists, or from uncertainty and fluctuation of mind, or even from a kind of fullness of learning, that they fell upon this opinion – have certainly advanced reasons for it that are not to be despised; but yet they have neither started from true principles nor rested in the just conclusion, zeal and affectation having carried them much too far.

The more ancient of the Greeks (whose writings are lost) took up with better judgment a position between these two extremes – between the presumption of pronouncing on everything, and the despair of comprehending anything; and though frequently and bitterly complaining of the difficulty of inquiry and the obscurity of things, and like impatient horses champing at the bit, they did not the less follow up their object and engage with nature, thinking (it seems) that this very question – viz., whether or not anything can be known – was to be settled not by arguing, but by trying. And yet they too, trusting entirely to the force of their understanding, applied no rule, but made everything turn upon hard thinking and perpetual working and exercise of the mind.

51 What does Bacon state is risked by people who "lay down the law of nature as a thing already searched out and understood" (line 2) ?

    A Inaccuracy.
    B Freedom of speech.
    C The impetus to refine knowledge.
    D The need for education.

52 Which THREE reasons does Bacon give for a person being of the opinion that "absolutely nothing can be known"(line 10)

I. The person is poorly educated.
II. The person is indecisive and unsure.
III. The person is overeducated.
IV. The person does not want to state his knowledge or theories.
V. The person resents philosophers.
VI. The person is afraid of his work being stolen or plagiarised.

    A I, III, V
    B II, III, V
    C I, II, III
    D I, IV, VI

53 What does Bacon mean by 'a position between these two extremes' (line 17)?

    A He believes we should aim for a compromise in all situations.
    B He is rejecting both all-encompassing theories and the idea that nothing can be known.
    C He is condemning extremism in matters of science and learning.
    D He is advocating a careful manner of making knowledge public.

54 Which TWO statements best describes the main purposes of Bacon's piece of writing.

I. To praise the ancient Greeks' methods.
II. To insult those who are too eager to define everything or claim that nothing can be defined.
III. To explain that in order to decide whether anything can be known the key is to keep trying.
IV. To express his anger over the narrow-mindedness of some scholars and thinkers.
V. To state his belief that people are too keen to jump to conclusions.

    A III, V
    B II, IV
    C I, II
    D I, III

UNIT 11 - Quotations

For each of the following quotations, select the phrase which is closest in meaning.

55 *If anyone believes that our smiles involve abandonment of the teaching of Marx, Engles and Lenin he deceives himself. Those who wait for that must wait until a shrimp learns to whistle. (Nikita Khrushchev, Speech in Moscow 1955).*

   A We will never do away with the teachings of Marx, Engels and Lenin.
   B It is ridiculous to think that we should stop the teaching of Marx, Engels and Lenin.
   C Everyone should follow the teachings of Marx, Engels and Lenin.
   D There is no reason for us to ignore the teachings of Marx, Engels and Lenin.

56 *All letters, methinks, should be free and easy as one's discourse, not studied as an oration, nor made up of hard words like a charm. (Dorothy Osborne, 1653)*

   A Letters should be written to be enjoyed.
   B Letters should be read many times to enjoy them.
   C Letters should be written like a conversation.
   D Letters should be written quickly without revisions.

57 *Science is made up of facts, as a house is made up of stones; but an accumulation of facts is no more a science than a heap of stones is a house. (Henri Poincare)*

   A Facts need a structure to be considered a science.
   B There is more to science than gathering facts together.
   C Science and houses have things in common.
   D Science is more complicated than house building.

58 *Gravitation cannot be held responsible for people falling in love. How on earth can you explain in terms of chemistry and physics so important a biological phenomenon as first love? Put your hand on a stove for a minute and it seems like an hour. Sit with that special girl for an hour and it seems like a minute. That's relativity. (Albert Einstein)*

    A Science is a good metaphor for life, even things it cannot explain.
    B Science can explain some things but not everything.
    C The theory of relativity can explain love.
    D Love cannot be described by science.

59 *One swallow does not make a summer. (Aristotle)*

    A Do not act immorally.
    B Do not make decisions based on false instinct.
    C Do not jump to conclusions.
    D Do not take things for granted.

60 *Perhaps the most valuable result of all education is the ability to make yourself do the thing you have to do, when it ought to be done, whether you like it or not; it is the first lesson that ought to be learned; and however early a man's training begins, it is probably the last lesson that he learns thoroughly. (Thomas H. Huxley)*

    A Becoming educated is very difficult no matter how early you start.
    B Developing discpline is key for the educated man.
    C The best outcome of education is being self-motivated.
    D Education is of no use if you cannot apply it.

61 *Science is the tool of the Western mind and with it more doors can be opened than with bare hands. It is part and parcel of our knowledge and obscures our insight only when it holds that the understanding given by it is the only kind there is. (Carl Jung)*

    A People of the West are better with science.
    B Science cannot explain everything.
    C Acting with scientific knowledge is more useful than acting without.
    D Science can breed arrogance.

Cartoons

UNIT 12 - Bush and Putin's Democracy Driving

The following cartoon pertains to the United States cultivating democracy around the world.

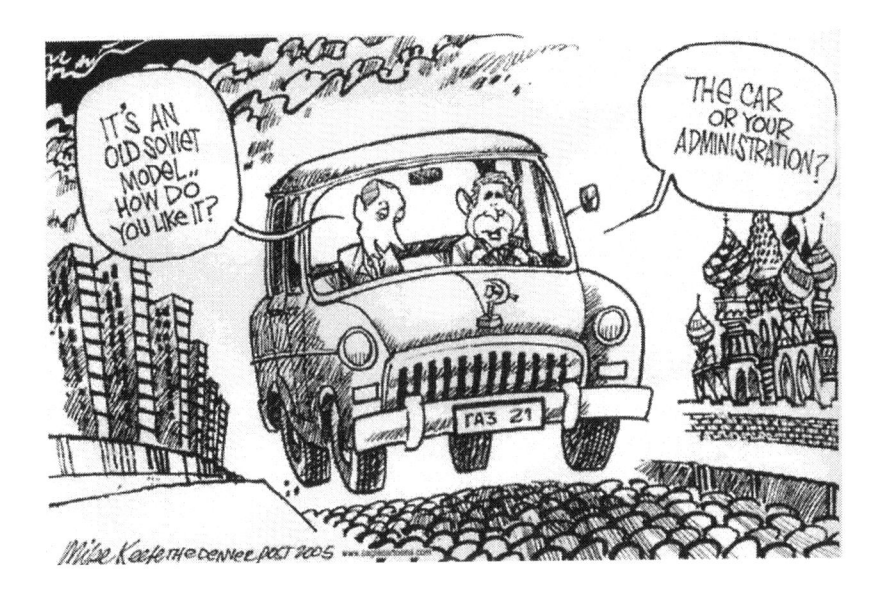

62 Bush's retort 'Your car or your administration?' implies that

   A the United States is still unclear about Putin's domestic policy.
   B the United States would like Russia to use the US as a role model of democracy.
   C under Putin, Russia remains a communist regime.
   D Putin is slow to remodel his administration along lines of a democratic government.

UNIT 13 - IVF

OLD FASHIONED LOVE STORY

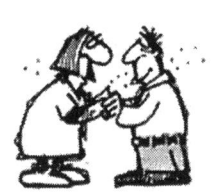

BOY MEETS GIRL

MODERN LOVE STORY

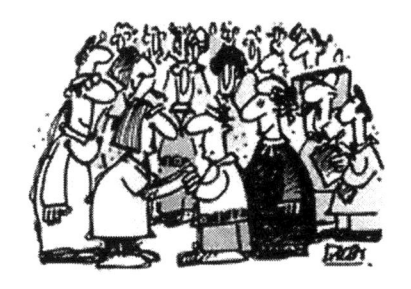

BOY MEETS GIRL, IVF MEDICAL TEAM, LEGAL TEAM, ETHICS COMMITTEE, TV CAMERA CREW ETC...

The above cartoon may be interpreted in more than one way. These are the four statements:

    I   Pregnancy is now a very public affair.
    II   The unnecessary and tedious road to conception.
    III The complexities of the technology of in-vitro fertilisation.
    IV The many-layered invasion into the private.

63 Which of these offer an overall opinion of in-vitro fertilisation?

    A Statement I only.
    B Statements II and III.
    C Statements I, III and IV.
    D Statement III only.

UNIT 14 - Long-term US energy policy

President Bush unveiled his energy policy which called for 'reliable, affordable and environmentally sound energy for America's future that at the same time meets the needs of today.'

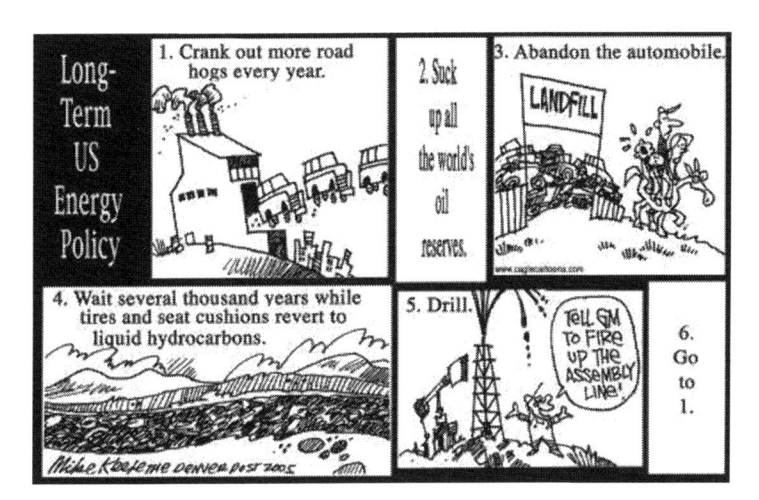

The above cartoon portrays Bush's government's plan in a highly negative light. These are four comments:

I   The US government's policy is an ad hoc one.
II The US government is a predator, buying up the world's reserves.
III The US government policy of balancing heavy energy needs and protecting the environment may be an unattainable goal.
IV It has no efficient policy to improve energy efficiency and conservation.

64 Which of the above statements are plausible interpretations of the cartoon?

   A I and II
   B I and IV
   C II and III
   D All of the above.

UNIT 15 - Another Food Pyramid

The cartoon below represents the USDA's creation of new customized version of the food pyramid.

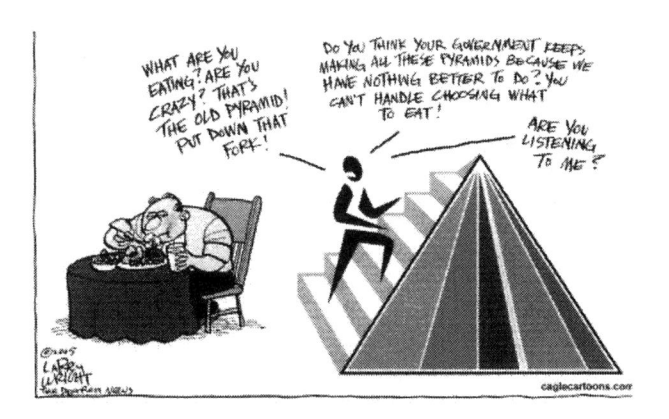

65 The 'old pyramid' refers to

    A an outdated idea
    B the 'one size fits all' food consumption guide
    C an unworkable system of nutrition
    D a nutrition disaster

66 'You can't handle choosing what to eat' implies that

    A individuals are not to be accountable for their own.
    B individuals have little knowledge of nutrition and diet.
    C individuals find it hard to follow a strict food guide.
    D the government must educate the public.

UNIT 16 - War On Terror

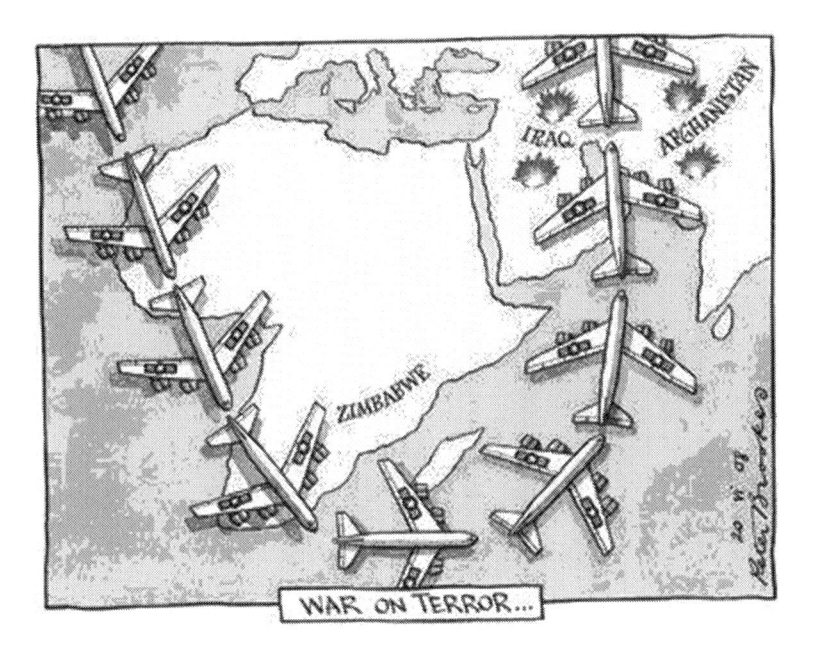

67 Which of the following phrases best describes the cartoonist's attitude to the situation in Zimbabwe?

    A It should be bypassed by violent Western forces.

    B The eyes of the world are upon Zimbabwe.

    C Zimbabwe is experiencing real terrorism.

    D Zimbabwe's problems will resolve themselves if left alone by foreigners.

68 What is the cartoonist's attitude to the wars on Iraq and Afghanistan?

    A They are equally pointless and undeserving of military action.

    B They are attracting too much military attention.

    C They are key platforms on which to fight against Terror.

    D They are detracting the attention of the world from other pertinent issues.

69 The caption 'War on Terror' aims to…

  A Point out that the three countries named are those which are currently suffering most severely from terrorism.
  B Highlight the irony of Iraq and Afghanistan attracting so much attention while Zimbabwe suffers from terrorism and is bypassed by forces.
  C Mock a hackneyed phrase which has lost its significance through over-use.
  D Blame interfering Western forces for the prevalence of terrorism.

70 Which of the following groups of words best describes the tone of this cartoon?

  A droll and innovative
  B political and uncompromising
  C solemn and conservative
  D angry and revolutionary

71 Which of these questions would best sum up the key message of the cartoon?

  A The idea of a war on terror is farcical, why does it persist?
  B What has Zimbabwe got to do with the War on Terror?
  C If it is really terrorism we are fighting, why are we bypassing what is happening in Zimbabwe?
  D Can't we leave Iraq and Afghanistan alone now that Zimbabwe needs our help?

UNIT 17 - Management

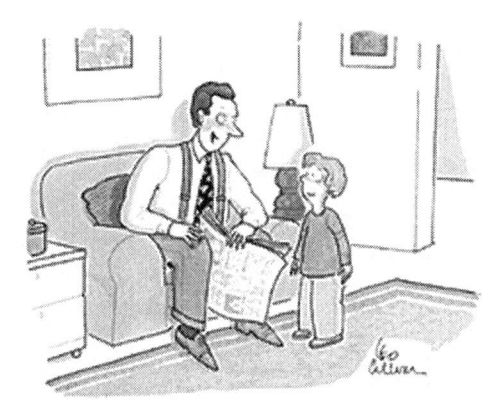

"Actually, Tommy, we're just about full-blooded management, except for your grandfather on your mom's side, who was one-quarter labor."

72 The humour in this cartoon arises from…

    A The idea of discussing complex issues with a child.

    B The idea of a child's ancestry being described in terms of the occupations of his forefathers.

    C The way in which the father dismisses the child's grandfather for being one-quarter labour.

    D The suggestion that the child has asked to know about his heritage.

73 There are a number of elements at work here. Read the following responses to the father in the cartoon.

> I. The father in the cartoon has poor parenting skills.
> II. The father is proud of his own family's management tradition.
> III. The father believes occupation to be what defines a family and it's future.
> IV. The father seems to reduce everything to terms of occupation.
> V. The father attempts to spread his poor judgement to his child.
> VI. The father is keen to limit his child's options for his future.
> VII. The father feels it is crucial for the son to understand his background.

Which THREE of the above statements are most correct.

    A I, II and IV
    B II, V and VI
    C II, IV and VII
    D III, VI and VII

Cartoons 45

UNIT 18 - Government Minister

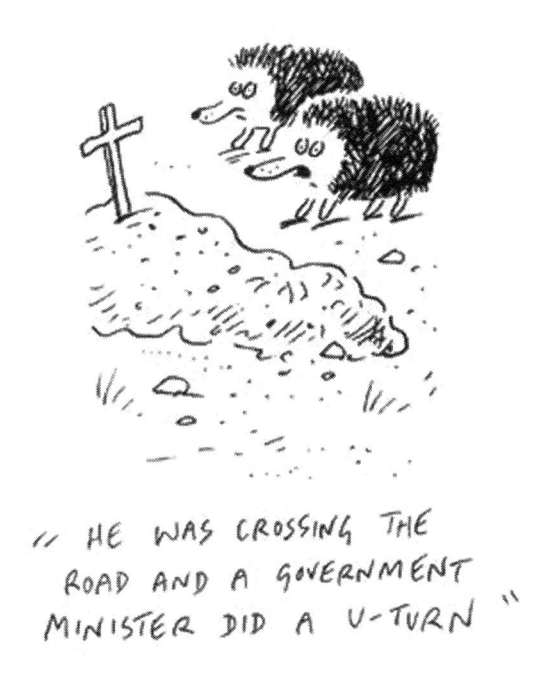

" HE WAS CROSSING THE ROAD AND A GOVERNMENT MINISTER DID A U-TURN "

74 What is the political message of this cartoon?

    A The government are acting irrationally.
    B Government ministers risk damage by changing their minds too often.
    C The government is a joke.
    D Governmental affairs are shady and far too difficult for the public to follow.

75 What is the cartoonist ridiculing?

    A The Government's public relations.
    B The public's attitude towards the Government.
    C The Government's decision-making process.
    D The solidarity of Government officials

76 The hedgehogs represent…

    A The average citizen, bemused by the Government's changing attitudes.
    B Those who stand up against the Government.
    C The victims of a badly run country.
    D Those damaged by changes in policy.

77 The cartoon suggests that the public's reaction to recent governmental decisions has been…

    A Out of proportion with the unimportant decisions they have been reacting to.
    B With hilarity and incredulity.
    C With growing anger and a sense of confusion.
    D With wonder and concern.

78 The humour of the cartoon…

    A highlights the imprudence of the Government.
    B ridicules recent Government decisions.
    C is offensive to those genuinely concerned about current Government policy.
    D points out the foolichness of those who are growing angry with the Government.

Cartoons 47

UNIT 19 - Business

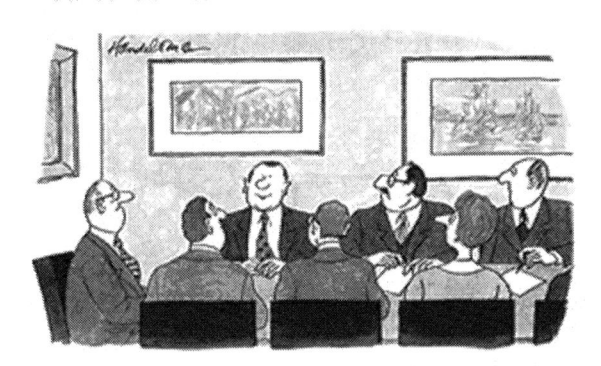

"You know what I think, folks? Improving technology isn't important. Increased profits aren't important. What's important is to be warm, decent human beings."

79 The humour in this cartoon is derived from…

    A The stupidity of the speaker
    B The expressions on the faces of the people reacting to the speaker
    C The unlikelihood of the speech
    D The idea of a business run on such principles as the speaker expresses

80 The message the cartoonist is expressing is closest to which of these phrases?

    A The idea of a business run with moral rather than financial objectives is ridiculous.
    B Modern businesses have a duty to act with integrity, even of it means sacrificing productivity.
    C Capitalism is not the uncompromising machine it is often accused of being.
    D Business people rarely employ warmth and humanity.

UNIT 20 - Same Sex

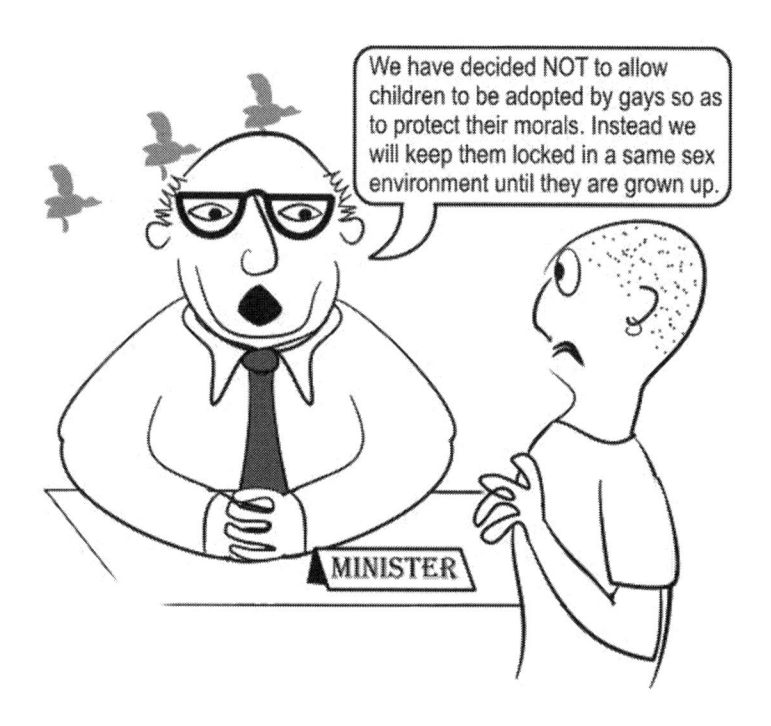

Speech bubble: We have decided NOT to allow children to be adopted by gays so as to protect their morals. Instead we will keep them locked in a same sex environment until they are grown up.

Nameplate: MINISTER

81 Which of the following phrases best describes the aim of this cartoon?

   A To encourage laughter at the predicament of the homosexual in prevailing society.
   B To highlight the magnitude of balanced family life.
   C To make it clear that the government has made an error of judgement.
   D To point out the irony of contemporary Governmental decisions.

82 The cartoonist most likely believes that homosexuality is...

   A not as pertinent to child-rearing as other concerns.
   B immoral and therefore damaging to a suggestible child.
   C not the government's concern.
   D not to be encouraged in the younger members of society.

83 The cartoon suggests that government ministers have an attitude which is…

    A old-fashioned and out-of-touch with modern society.
    B potentially dangerous to young people.
    C unfair to children's homes which are overcrowded and financially stretched.
    D poorly thought-out and flawed in an extremely obvious way.

84 Which of the following best describes how the cartoonist feels about children being brought up in various environments?

    A A same-sex couple is more damaging to a child than a children's home.
    B A children's home is more damaging to a child than a same-sex couple.
    C Government Ministers should not be the ones to decide where a child grows up.
    D A same-sex couple is a better environment for a child than a being locked away in a children's home.

85 The tone of the cartoon is mainly…

    A comical and flippant - a joke.
    B satirical and sarcastic - a parody.
    C world-weary and pessimistic - a warning.
    D politically aware and activist - a message.

UNIT 21 - Boyfriend

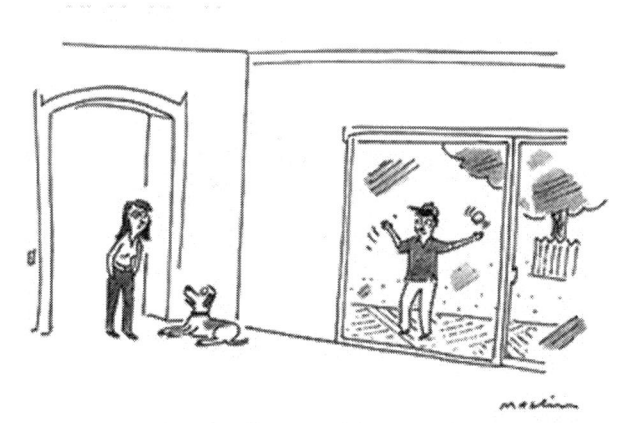

"You're the one who wanted a boyfriend—you play with him."

86 The persona of the dog in this cartoon...

    A Is a hyperbolic representation of a typical dog's personality
    B Is in charge of the household, dominating the woman.
    C Is placed in role-reversal situation with the boyfriend for humorous effect.
    D Is humorous because he owns the boyfriend as a pet rather than being owned.

87 The concept behind the cartoon is that...

    A Men are surplus to a woman's requirements nowadays.
    B The woman and the dog have acquired a boyfriend much as a couple would acquire a pet.
    C The dog is a more valuable companion than a partner.
    D The woman has very quickly grown tired of her new boyfriend.

UNIT 22 - Beach

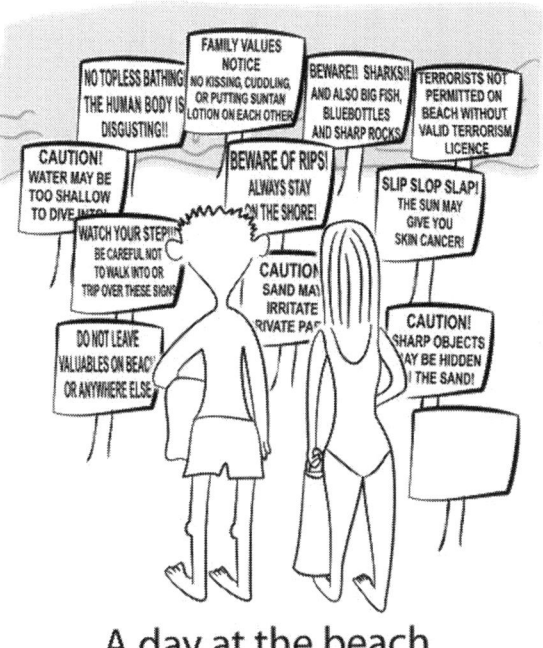

A day at the beach

88 The cartoon's key suggestion is that…

    A people have no freedom nowadays.
    B health and safety are important issues in the modern world.
    C guidance on beaches hampers the public's enjoyment.
    D restrictions on beaches have become over-the-top and ridiculous.

89 Which of these wider concerns does the cartoon address?

    A over-cautiousness, the 'nanny state'.
    B paranoia, natural disaster.
    C the public's fear of crime, health 'scares'.
    D health management, compensation claims.

90 The tone of the cartoon is mainly…

    A sardonic, sharp.
    B puerile, inane.
    C tense, strained.
    D radical, uncompromising.

91 The attitude of the cartoonist towards censorship in Australia is…

    A She feels oppressed by it.
    B She feels it is detrimental to the country.
    C She feels the public are irritated by it.
    D She feels it is outlandish.

92 The signs in the cartoon are…

    A Symbolic of real fears the public feel when visiting a beach
    B Completely imagined by the creator for humorous effect
    C Hyperbolic representations of the types of restrictions seen on beaches
    D Representative of general censorship in Australian society which stifles personal freedom.

UNIT 23 - Conversation

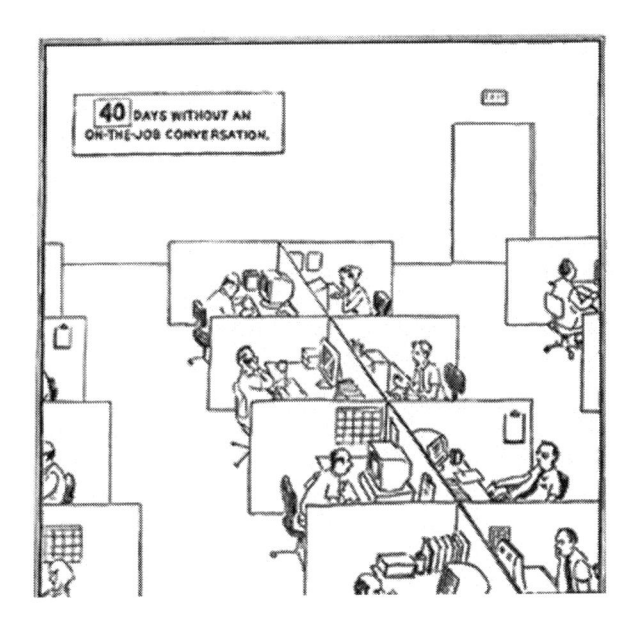

93 This cartoon implies a number of meanings. Read the following responses.

I. Office work can be isolating.
II. The practice of forbidding conversations in the workplace is demoralising.
III. Office politics can lead to a cold environment.
IV. A dedicated workplace has no need for on-the-job conversations.
V. Offices tend to view a quiet, insulated workforce as a good thing.

Which of the following options describes the responses which are correct.

    A I and II.
    B III and V
    C I and V
    D II and IV

94 The humour in the cartoon arises from…

   A The idea of such a soulless workplace, an exaggerated version of a typical office.
   B Replacing a typical measurement of success sign on the wall with one championing lack of conversation.
   C The blandness of the prolonged silence.
   D Then impossibility of a workplace which can avoid on-the-job conversations.

UNIT 24 - Petrol

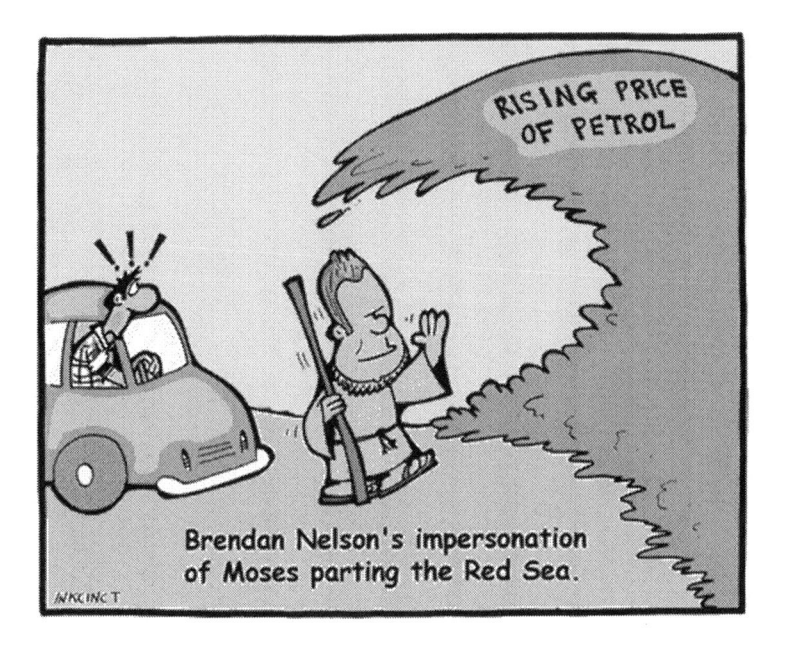

Brendan Nelson's impersonation of Moses parting the Red Sea.

RISING PRICE OF PETROL

95 The implication of the cartoon is that Nelson's claim that he has the ability to stem the cost of petrol is…

  A being proved correct.
  B being proved wrong.
  C an over confident assumption.
  D a bare-faced lie.

96 The cartoon portrays Nelson as…

  A A self assured yet over-confident leader, in control but threatened with disaster.
  B A successful and powerful leader, staving off threats to the public he represents.
  C A blasphemous and dangerous person, with a delusion of power.
  D A foolish and ridiculous figure, casting himself as a social miracle worker.

97 Rising petrol costs are shown by the cartoon to be...

    A mostly avoidable if appropriate action is taken with caution.
    B frustrating to the public who have to deal with a worsening financial climate.
    C an inevitable occurrence - a potential disaster which we cannot now avoid.
    D a moral issue, one which requires proper guidance.

98 Which of the following phrases is most likely to be advice given by the cartoonist to the public?

    A Don't panic about rising fuel prices!
    B Trust Nelson - he has things under control!
    C Fuel prices are spiralling out of control!
    D Be wary of false promises!

99 What does the cartoon suggest is a risk to the Australian motorist?

    A burgeoning fuel costs causing widespread financial hardship.
    B being let down as a result of trusting Nelson's claims.
    C rising sea levels due to climate change causing havoc.
    D Nelson's show of power causing unwanted Governmental change.

UNIT 25 - Ritual

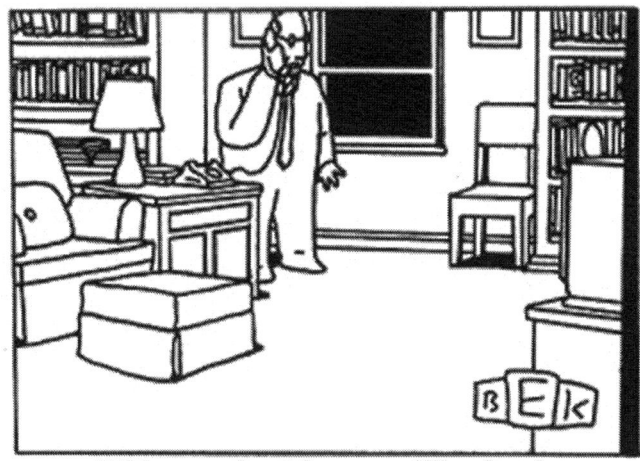

"I'd love to, but I have a million lonely ritualistic things I need to do."

100   This cartoon makes a number of implications. Read the following responses.

   I.   The cartoon is a comment on modern life
   II.   The male character is a representation of modern isolation.
   III. The cartoon's main purpose is to encourage laughter at the plight of modern man.
   IV.   There is a sense of chaos in the world the cartoon conjures up.
   V.   There is a strong sense of irony at the man's rejection of company in favour of loneliness.
   VI.   The cartoon is a scathing warning against the rejection of social contact.

Which THREE statements are most correct?

   A I, IV and V
   B I, II and VI
   C II, III and V
   D I, II and V

101 The cartoon's tone is most like which of these phrases?

   A   a sense of dystopia and disturbing realism
   B   depressing and confusing for no reason
   C   sharply observed comedic work
   D   a social comment intended to repulse.

Poetry

UNIT 26 - Gwendolyn Brooks "Kitchenette Building"

Kitchenette Building

We are things of dry hours and the involuntary plan,   1
Grayed in and gray. "Dream" mate, a giddy sound, not strong
Like "rent", "feeding a wife", "satisfying a man".

But could a dream sent up through onion fumes   5
Its white and violet, fight with fried potatoes
And yesterday's garbage ripening in the hall,
Flutter or sing an aria down these rooms,

Even if we were willing to let it in,   10
Had time to warm it, keep it very clean,
Anticipate a message, let it begin?

We wonder. But not well! Not for a minute!
Since number five is out of the bathroom now,   15
We think of lukewarm water, hope to get in it

Gwendolyn Brooks

102 The 'we' in the poem refers to

    A the parents
    B the children
    C women
    D husbands

103 'We are things of dry hours and involuntary plans' refers to

   A the emptiness of the speaker's life.
   B the commitment of the persona in the poem
   C the impromptu roles that the 'we' in the poem have to play.
   D the functional aspects of daily life.

104 The effect of personifying 'dream' is

   A to help the reader see 'dream' as a human and concrete part of the poem.
   B to make it come true.
   C to establish a sense of hope in the lives of the family
   D to ensure that something so elusive can be felt.

105 The second stanza reveals feelings of

   A despair
   B hope
   C frustration
   D desperation

106 The poem is about

   A the daily grind of existence.
   B poverty and dreams.
   C women's lot.
   D women's roles.

UNIT 27 - Louis Macniece "Song"

Song

The sunlight on the garden   1
Hardens and grow cold.
We cannot cage the minute
Within its net of gold:
When all is told   5
We cannot beg for pardon.

Our freedom as free lances
Advances towards its end;
The earth compels, upon it   10
Sonnets and birds descend:
And soon, my friend,
We shall have no time for dances.

The sky was good for flying   15
Defying the church bells
And every evil iron
Siren and what it tells:
The earth compels,
We are dying, Egypt, dying   20

And not expecting pardon,
Hardened in heart anew,
But glad to have sat under
Thunder and rain with you,   25
And grateful too
For sunlight on the garden.

Louis Macniece

107 In the first stanza, the persona in the poem is communicating to the reader

   A his coming to terms with the realization that a certain stage of life cannot be prolonged.
   B about a broken relationship.
   C news of his imminent death.
   D that all good things come to an end.

108 The second stanza beginning 'Our freedom as free lances............' means that

   A the persona regrets the futile years of youth
   B he is grateful that every phase of life is closing.
   C age has its place and we have to accept it.
   D the freedom of youth, when everything is possible, is passing.

109 The imagery of life as a fighter pilot in the lines beginning:
'The sky was good for flying', 'Defying the church bells..........' brings to mind the idea of

   A an escape from a restrictions and conventions.
   B the sky's the limit.
   C the vastness of youth's ambitions.
   D the dynamism and heroics of youth.

110 'The earth compels' implies a certain sense of

   A anger.
   B wistfulness.
   C inevitability.
   D resentment.

111 The poem concludes with a feeling of

   A gratitude.
   B nostalgia.
   C acceptance.
   D all of the above.

UNIT 28 - Humbert Wolfe "The Grey Squirrel"

The Grey Squirrel

Like a small grey   1
coffee-pot,
sits the squirrel.
He is not

All he should be,   6
kills by dozens
trees, and eats
his red-brown cousins.

The keeper, on the   11
other hand, who
shot him, is
a Christian, and

loves his enemies,   16
which shows
the squirrel was not
one of them.

Humbert Wolfe

112 The effect of the opening simile, in relation to the whole poem, is

    A very cute
    B very disarming.
    C very charming.
    D very appropriate.

113 The grey squirrel is 'not all that he should be' because

   A he is a creature with a hidden agenda.
   B he is small and thus very pernicious.
   C he eats his fellow rodents.
   D he is not man's natural enemy.

114 The keeper is a representative of

   A trigger-happy hunters.
   B the Christian community.
   C the Christian concept of 'love thine enemies'.
   D systematic squirrel control.

115 The first twist in the poem is the idea that

   A the Christian keeper should be as brutal as the squirrel.
   B grey squirrels are not our idealized creatures.
   C humans err.
   D there is a fracture between principle and practice.

116 The second twist in the poem is

   A gamekeepers cannot have squeamish consciences.
   B the conundrum of conservation.
   C the unexpected lack of charity of a Christian.
   D the Christian is not our idealized version of a Christian.

117 The poem is a sharp exposé of

   A the hypocrisy of religion.
   B illogical reasoning.
   C the ethics of culling.
   D the dilemma of conservation.

UNIT 29 - Linda Pastan "Ethics"

Ethics

In ethics class so many years ago
our teacher asked this question every fall:
if there were a fire in a museum
which would you save, a Rembrandt painting
or an old woman who hadn't many
years left anyhow? Restless on hard chairs
caring little for pictures or old age
we'd opt on e year for lir, the next for art
and always half-heartedly. Sometimes
the woman borrowed my grandmother's face
leaving her usual kitchen to wonder
some drafty, half-imagined museum.
One year, feeling clever, I replied
why not let the woman decide herself?
Linda, the teacher would report, eshews
the burden of responsibility.
This fall in a real museum I stand
before a real Rembrandt, old woman,
or nearly so, myself. The colours
within this frame are darker than autumn,
darker even than winter - the browns of earth
though earth's most radiant elements burn
through the canvas. I know now that woman
and painting and season are almost one
and all beyond saving for children.

Linda Pastan

118 The speaker in this poem is

    A a young child.
    B an older woman.
    C the ethics teacher.
    D the grandmother.

119 The speaker's and her classmates' attitude to 'pictures' and 'old age' was

    A indifferent
    B imaginative
    C uncomprehending
    D disinterested

120 The class answered the teacher's question 'half-heartedly' because

    A it was too difficult.
    B the teacher expected a clear choice.
    C the class was too young.
    D the situation was not "real"

121 The subject of this poem is

    A value judgments
    B whether life or art is more valuable
    C issue of moral responsibility
    D time

122 The meaning of the poem is contributed mainly by

    A the question posed by the teacher each fall.
    B the remark by the teacher about Linda's shunning responsibility.
    C the contrast in settings, situations and characters.
    D the real Rembrandt and the real Museum.

123 The conclusion of the speaker, reflected in the line "and all beyond saving my children" is

    A the futility of teaching ethics to the very young
    B the fact that what one saves is crucial but not simple
    C the question of shifting values
    D the time is inexorable

UNIT 30 - Dame Mary Gilmore "Eve Song"

Eve-Song

I span and Eve span   1
A thread to bind the heart of man;
But the heart of man was a wandering thing
That came and went with little to bring:
Nothing he minded what we made,   5
As here he loitered, and there he stayed.
I span and Eve span
A thread to bind the heart of man;
But the more we span the more we found
It wasn't his heart but ours we bound.   10
For children gathered about our knees:
The thread was a chain that stole our ease.
And one of us learned in our children's eyes
That more than man was love and prize.
But deep in the heart of one of us lay   15
A root of loss and hidden dismay.

He said he was strong. He had no strength
But that which comes of breadth and length.
He said he was fond. But his fondness proved 20
The flame of an hour when he was moved.
He said he was true. His truth was but
A door that winds could open and shut.

And yet, and yet, as he came back,   25
Wandering in from the outward track,
We held our arms, and gave him our breast,
As a pillowing place for his head to rest.
I span and Eve span,
A thread to bind the heart of man!   30

Dame Mary Gilmore

124 Line 1 is significant because…

   A the poet is talking about all women, from Eve the first woman to herself.
   B she is pointing out how much work women have to do.
   C she is referring to how women work together.
   D the poet wants the reader to know how hard she works.

125 Line 12, 'The thread was a chain that stole our ease' suggests that…

   A the work of the women is too difficult.
   B work did not make the women as happy as they thought it would.
   C having children bound the women to a difficult life.
   D life has been full of disappointment for the women.

126 The second stanza (beginning with line 18) is mainly a list of…

   A the broken promises of men.
   B the lies which men have told.
   C mistakes which men have made.
   D ways in which men have disappointed women.

127 'His truth was but / A door that winds could open and shut'. The meaning of lines 22-23 can best be summed up by which phrase?

   A 'He told me lies'
   B 'He did not understand how to be honest'
   C 'He subtly tried to trick me at every opportunity'
   D 'His honesty was inconstant'

128 Reread the last section of the poem. This section shows…

   A that the women and men are a comfort to each other.
   B that whatever their faults the women are there for the men.
   C that there is real love between the men and women.
   D that the men really are bound to the women.

129 The main theme of this poem is…

    A the love between a married couple.
    B how women have a tougher life than men.
    C the difficulties of the life of a married woman.
    D how men treat women poorly.

UNIT 31 - Percy Bysshe Shelley "Ozymandias"

Ozymandias

I met a traveller from an antique land   1
Who said: "Two vast and trunkless legs of stone
Stand in the desert. Near them on the sand,
Half sunk, a shattered visage lies, whose frown
And wrinkled lip and sneer of cold command   5
Tell that its sculptor well those passions read
Which yet survive, stamped on these lifeless things,
The hand that mocked them and the heart that fed.
And on the pedestal these words appear:
`My name is Ozymandias, King of Kings: 10
Look on my works, ye mighty, and despair!'
Nothing beside remains. Round the decay
Of that colossal wreck, boundless and bare,
The lone and level sands stretch far away.   14

Percy Bysshe Shelley

130 In line 4, the 'shattered visage' is…

    A The face of Ozymandias.
    B A stone carving of Ozymandias.
    C The face of the traveller.
    D The traveller's vision of a face in the sand.

131 To whom does the poem refer in line 8 'The hand that mocked them and the heart that fed'.

    A The narrator of the poem
    B The poet himself.
    C Ozymandias.
    D A sculptor.

132 How does the poet most want the reader to think of Ozymandias?

   A As a great historical leader and King.
   B As a traveller's vision.
   C As a once-great man.
   D As a subject for the sculptor's art.

133 Which of the following phrases most fully describes the poem's message?

   A Everyone must die someday.
   B Even stone will one day wear away.
   C The desert is inhospitable to men.
   D Man's power on earth is only temporary.

134 The last 5 lines of the poem mostly describe…

   A the sadness of Ozymandias' fall from power.
   B the desolation of the desert.
   C the irony of Ozymandias' claim as King of Kings.
   D the loneliness of the traveller in the desert.

135 What impression are we given of the sculptor?

   A That his work was not able to stand the test of time well.
   B That he was able to read and capture the expression of his subject.
   C That he has destroyed his own sculpture.
   D That he was mightier than Ozymandias.

UNIT 32 - G. Essex Evans "The Women On The West"

The Women of the West

They left the vine-wreathed cottage and the mansion on the hill, 1
The houses in the busy streets where life is never still,
The pleasures of the city, and the friends they cherished best;
For love they faced the wilderness - the Women of the West.

The roar, and rush, and fever of the city died away, 6
And the old-time joys and faces-they were gone for many a day,
In their place the lurching coach-wheel, or the creaking bullock-chains,
O'er the everlasting sameness of the never-ending plains.

In the slab-built, zinc-roofed homestead of some lately taken run, 11
In the tent beside the bankment of a railway just begun,
In the huts on new selections, in the camps of man's unrest,
On the frontiers of the Nation, live the Women of the West.

The red sun robs their beauty and, in weariness and pain, 16
The slow years steal the nameless grace that never comes again;
And there are hours men cannot soothe, and words men cannot say
The nearest woman's face may be a hundred miles away.

The wide bush holds the secrets of their longing and desire, 21
When the white stars in reverence light their holy altar fires,
And silence, like the touch of God, sinks deep into the breast-
Perchance He hears and understands the Women of the West.

Well have we held our father's creed. No call has passed us by. 26
We faced and fought the wilderness, we sent our sons to die.
And we have hearts to do and dare, and yet, o'er all the rest,
The hearts that made the Nation were the Women of the West 29

G. Essex Evans

136 Which THREE of the following statements best describe the problems the poet tells us the women encounter in their lives in the West.

I. The women were separated for a long time from people they once knew.
II. The journey to the West often made the women become ill.
III. The women were separated from their husbands for long periods of time.
IV. The women were mistreated by their men.
V. The women lose their looks because of the sun and the harshness of time spent in the West.
VI. The women feel angry about their suffering.
VII. The women miss the company of other females who are often far away.
VIII. The women often have to work for long periods of time without gratitude.

A I, V, VII
B II, III, VI
C I, IV, VIII
D II, III, VII

137 What was the reason for women to move to the West?

A In search of a better life.
B To get away from the cities.
C For the love of their men.
D For the adventure.

138 Which of the following statements best summarises what the poet means by line 29 'The hearts that made the Nation were the Women of the West'?

A The Women of the West are people to be proud of.
B The strength of our nation is founded on the Women of the West.
C Women of the West are our ancestors.
D We owe our love and respect to the Women of the West.

139 What phrase best describes the women in the poem?

    A healthy and adventurous
    B hard-working and content
    C resilient and brave
    D lonely and mistreated

140 What is the purpose of this poem? Select the phrase which best describes the poet's intentions.

    A To pay tribute to the Women of the West.
    B To express sadness at what these women went through.
    C To help the reader learn about Australian history.
    D To make the reader feel anger at how poorly treated the women were.

UNIT 33 - John Keats "The Human Seasons"

The Human Seasons

Four Seasons fill the measure of the year;   1
There are four seasons in the mind of man:
He has his lusty Spring, when fancy clear
Takes in all beauty with an easy span:
He has his Summer, when luxuriously   5
Spring's honied cud of youthful thought he loves
To ruminate, and by such dreaming high
Is nearest unto heaven: quiet coves
His soul has in its Autumn, when his wings
He furleth close; contented so to look   10
On mists in idleness--to let fair things
Pass by unheeded as a threshold brook.
He has his Winter too of pale misfeature,
Or else he would forego his mortal nature.   14

John Keats

141 What is the main theme of the poem?

   A The four seasons - Spring, Summer, Autumn and Winter.
   B The passage of time.
   C The change in a persons mind as they age.
   D The fragility and shortness of human life.

142 Which of the following phrases best describes the 'Spring' of a man's mind according to the poem?

   A The man is appreciative of beauty.
   B The man is imaginative and relaxed.
   C The man feels lustful.
   D The man has many thoughts in his mind.

143 Which of the following phrases best describes the 'Summer' of a man's mind according to the poem?

    A He is at the most busy time of his life.
    B He enjoys thinking over the sweetness of his youth.
    C He spends his time dreaming.
    D He looks forward to the pleasures of being older.

144 Which of the following phrases best describes the 'Autumn' of a man's mind according to the poem?

    A The man is happy to watch the world go by.
    B The man is saddened by passing time.
    C The man becomes lazy.
    D The man is tired out by life.

145 Which of the following phrases best describes the 'Winter' of a man's mind according to the poem?

    A The winter of his mind is unremarkable but necessary.
    B The winter of his mind is an unproductive time.
    C In the winter of his life the man is miserable.
    D The winter of his life is boring.

146 Which phrase has the closest meaning to the line 'to let fair things / Pass by unheeded as a threshold brook'?

    A To let opportunities pass by without taking advantage of them.
    B To allow beautiful thoughts flow effortlessly through the mind.
    C To ignore things which are fair.
    D To think of beautiful natural things - like a stream.

Sociology

UNIT 34 - Daniel Bell "Modernisn, postmodernism and the decline of moral order"

PASSAGE from 'Modernisn, postmodernism and the decline of moral order': Daniel Bell

Culture and Society Alexander and Seidman

So long as work and wealth had a religious sanction, they possessed a transcendental justification. But when that ethic eroded, there was a loss of legitimation, for the pursuit of wealth alone is not a calling that justifies itself. As Schumpeter once shrewdly remarked: The stock exchange is a poor substitute for the Holy Grail. The central point is that - at first, for the advanced social groups, the intelligentsia and the educated social classes, and later for the middle class itself - the legitimations of social behavior passed from religion to modernist culture. And with it here was a shift in emphasis from "character," which is the unity of moral codes and disciplined purpose, to an emphasis on "personality," which is the enhancement of self through the compulsive search for individual differentiation. In brief, not work but the "life style" became the source of satisfaction and criterion for desirable behavior in the society.
Yet paradoxically, the life style that became the imago of the free self was not that of the businessman, expressing himself through his "dynamic drive," but that of the artist defying the conventions of the society.
And, as I have tried to show, increasingly, it is the artist who begins to dominate the audience, and to impose his judgment as to what is to be desired and bought. The paradox is completed when the bourgeois ethic, having collapsed in the society, finds few defenders in the culture (do any writers defend any institutions?) and Modernism, as an attack on orthodoxy, has triumphed and become the regnant orthodoxy of the day.

Any tension creates its own dialectic. Since the market is where social structure and culture cross, what has happened is that in the last fifty years the economy has been geared to producing the life styles paraded by the culture. Thus, not only has there been a contradiction between the realms, but that tension has produced a further contradiction within the economic realm itself. In the world of capitalist enterprise, the nominal ethos in the spheres of production and organization is still one of work, delayed gratification, career orientation, devotion to the enterprise, yet, on the marketing side, the sale of goods, packaged in the glossy images of glamour and sex, promotes a hedonistic way of life whose promise is the voluptuous gratification of the lineaments of desire. The consequence of this contradiction, as I put it in these pages, is that a corporation fields its people being straight by day and swingers by night.

What has happened in society in the last fifty years — as a result of the erosion of the religious ethic and the increase in discretionary income — is that the culture has taken the initiative in promoting change, and the economy has been geared to meeting these new wants.

In this respect, there has been a significant reversal in the historical pattern of social change. During the rise of capitalism - in the "modernization" of any traditional society - one could more readily change the economic structure of a society: by forcing people off the land into factories, by imposing a new rhythm and discipline of work, by using brutal means or incentives (e.g. the theory of interest as the reward for "abstinence" from consumption) to raise capital. But the "superstructure" - the patterns of family life, the attachments to religion and authority, the received ideas that shaped people's perceptions of a social reality – was more stubbornly resistant to change.

Today, by contrast, it is the economic structure that is the more difficult to change. Within the enterprise, the heavy bureaucratic layers reduce flexible adaptation, while union rules inhibit the power of management to control the assignment of jobs. In the society, the economic enterprise is subject to the challenges of various veto groups (e.g. on the location of plants or the use of the environment) and subject more and more to regulation by government.

But in the culture, fantasy reigns almost unconstrained. The media are geared to feeding new images to people, to unsettling traditional conventions, and the highlighting of aberrant and quirky behavior which becomes images for other to imitate. The traditional is stodgy, and the "orthodox" institutions such as family and church are on the defensive about their inability to change. Yet if capitalism has been routinized, Modernism has been trivialized. After all, how often can it continue to shock if there is nothing shocking left? If experiment is the norm, how original can anything new be? And like all bad history, Modernism has repeated its end, once in the popgun outbursts of Futurism and Dadaism, the second time in the phosphorescent parodies of Pop paintings and the mindless minimalism of conceptual art.

147 The passage, as a whole, is a critique of

   A the lifestyle of conspicuous consumption
   B the inadequacy and immoral character of modernist culture.
   C the loss of a rational and moral criteria for behaviour in modern society.
   D the role of political and economic structures.

148 "The stock exchange is a poor substitute for the Holy Grail." This quotation is used by the writer to underscore his point that

   A the present motivator of behaviour is sole pursuit of wealth.
   B the discipline of work is lost in favour of "the quick buck".
   C the imperative for wealth creation has eroded society's common moral core.
   D the imperative for wealth creation is the new Holy Grail.

149 The writer says that modern society is driven by

   A career orientation
   B moral codes.
   C ceaseless search for lifestyle
   D purposelessness

150 Bell states: "It is the economic structure that is more difficult to change". His reasons are:

   A Bureaucracies and lobby groups rule this realm.
   B Managements are subject to union regulations.
   C Tight controls are kept on it by government.
   D All of the above.

151 In the lines "The media are geared to feeding new images to people............", it is understood that

   A the impact of the media is negative.
   B the media promote counter cultures.
   C the media attacts tradition.
   D the media are the new forms of cultural communication.

152 According to the passage, modern man is dominated by

   A fascination with the shock of the new.
   B rebellion against established religion
   C the individual self as a measure of satisfaction.
   D efficiency and productivity.

153 Bell's main theme is that, in attacking established norms, the new culture of modernist society is

   A undermining itself
   B contradicting itself by establishing non-conformity as the norm
   C condoning anarchism
   D trivializing all values

Australian

UNIT 35 - Chloe Hooper "A Child's Book of True Crime"

Read the extract from *A Child's Book of True Crime* by Chloe Hooper and answer the questions which follow.

I looked out the window. Slowly, the mothers were gathering in the playground. There was an old ship's bell under the jacaranda. In five minutes, at half-past three, it would ring and all the children would run outside. I moved around the room trying to seem natural and bright to those on the other side of the glass. Most of the mothers had sensible hair and sensible shoes. Except for Veronica. Pale Veronica with skin that held the light. Through the window, I'd long studied her looks; her trademark red lipstick confusing, or perhaps accentuating, all the orchid delicacy she had going for her.

Turning back to the class, it was difficult to muster composure. Veronica and I were initially quite cordial, but after reading her book, I walked around my house as if visible from every angle; suddenly the walls were made of eyes. Then at night, late, the telephone started ringing.

If it came down to some sort of tussle, I would obviously have the advantage of youth; she was pushing 40 and I was at least 15 years her junior. Plus she was so thin, very thin and graceful; if I wasn't badly stunned I could easily outbulk her... Veronica's main advantage would be strategy. Ever since she was young she'd read these parlour detective stories where crime is so pristine, always conforming to a trusted formula: after the stableboy-with-ringworm finds the deceased under a pile of hay, everything is conducted in a most urbane fashion; interrogations take place during high tea. When the murderer breaks down and politely confesses, they all have gin and tonics on the lawn.

One day Veronica had had I-could-do-that syndrome. Always canny, she discovered true crime sold better than fiction - and who could make this stuff up? A small-town American football star murders local girls using soda pop bottles. A wealthy British doctor kills his wife and her maid; then cuts off their identifying characteristics: fingertips, eyeballs (the maid had a bad squint), and teeth (his wife's were bucked).

154 Throughout the extract, the narrator gives the impression of being mainly…

   A jealous and paranoid
   B anxious and obsessive
   C scholarly and unhappy
   D confused and worried

155 What are the occupations of the women in the extract?

   A student and teacher.
   B they are both writers.
   C teacher and housewife/mother.
   D teacher and writer.

156 Which of the following descriptions best describes the character of Veronica?

   A intelligent, thoughtful and motherly.
   B striking, interesting and accomplished.
   C dainty, successful and tactical.
   D beautiful, talented and threatening.

157 'Most of the mothers had sensible hair and sensible shoes'. What is the purpose of line 5?

   A To describe the type of mothers the narrator can see.
   B To show the narrator's attention to detail.
   C To provide a contrast between most of the mothers and Veronica.
   D To show how different the narrator is from the mothers.

158 Read from line 18 'Ever since she was young she'd read these parlour detective stories…' to line 23, 'gin and tonics on the lawn' What is the point to this paragraph?

    A The paragraph is describing a particular story which Veronica read when she was young.
    B This paragraph describes a clichéd story typical of the types of stories Veronica read when she was young.
    C This paragraph is making a joke of the kind of stories Veronica writes.
    D This paragraph is describing exactly the kind of story which Veronica loves and the narrator hates.

159 What type of stories does Veronica write?

    A Easily-resolved mysteries.
    B Accounts of real-life crimes.
    C Fictional stories based on real murders.
    D Many different kinds of stories.

UNIT 36 - Paul Kelly "The Changes, The Challenges, The Choices For Australia"

Read this extract from *The changes, the challenges, the choices for Australia* by Paul Kelly and answer the questions which follow.

Australians tend to take the past for granted, worry about the present and postpone the future. If this is right, it might be the virtue of a still young country. But we take too little note of political history, seeing war, military history and sport as closest to our identity.

I think there is a bigger market for Australian history than most publishing houses would believe.

Angle and promotion are, of course, the keys. In the 1970s we found on the late National Times a tremendous interest among our readers in contemporary Australian history. In the 1990s as Editor-in-Chief of The Australian, I devoted considerable resources to historical themes–a tribute to the 1950s, a commemoration of the 50th anniversary of John Curtin's death, an historical special on the paper's 30th birthday, the Beatles' trip to Australia, the post-war immigration program, the 25th anniversary of that famous year 1968, the Republic debate and many others. These themes were popular because they worked for the paper in circulation terms, disproving the view of those who dismissed contemporary history as a point of genuine interest. A spin off was that we involved prominent Australian academics writing at length for the newspaper.

As we approach the centenary of Federation the issue of what it means and how it should be commemorated will press upon us. Federation, I think, has had a bad press for too long. It is an idea and a movement which is more powerful than is commonly depicted.

160 For what reason does the writer discuss his time as editor-in-chief for The Australian?

   A To establish his credentials.
   B To back up his claim that there is a demand for historical knoweldge.
   C To promote newspapers as a means of increasing interest in history.
   D To explain his own interest in history.

161 Which one of the following options best sums up the writers attitude towards political history?

   A It is more important than other types of history.
   B It is not given as much space in newspapers as it was in previous decades.
   C It will become more important as time goes on.
   D It involves a more academic style of writing.

162 Select the phrase that best describes advice that the article gives to the Australian citizen.

   A Ignore claims that history is inconsequential.
   B Increase demand for political history.
   C Readdress your sense of identity.
   D Celebrate the successes of the past.

163 Which of these phrases best describes the Kelly's opinion of himself?

   A He feels he has valuable experience he should share.
   B He believes he knows more about the relevant issues than other experts.
   C He is prepared to exaggerate in order to be believed.
   D He feels he is obligated to promote social change.

164 Which of the following seems most important for Kelly to communicate?

   A That interest in contemporary history is thriving.
   B That people are in danger of becoming ignorant of their own heritage.
   C That as time passes people will come to value their cultural history more.
   D That political and contemporary history are crucially important.

165 Taking into consideration the tone of the article, which of the following best describes how line 1/2, 'Australians tend to take the past for granted, worry about the present and postpone the future' is intended to be received?

   A A witty generalisation.
   B A patronising affront.
   C A light-hearted throwaway comment.
   D A derogatory joke.

UNIT 37 - Robert Hughes "The Fatal Shore"

This passage is taken from Robert Hughes's *The Fatal Shore: The Epic of Australia's Founding.*

THE FANTASY of escape to China was one of the obsessive images of early transportation. Yellow girls and tea, opium and silk, queer-looking blue bridges and willows just like the ones on plates; and surcease from the hoe, the iron, the roasting sunlight and the dumb ache of hunger. For this, not a few of the "deluded Irish" died of fatigue, thirst or the spears of blacks. Their crow-pecked remains, with a rag of government slops and a rusty basil still around them, would be found in the bush between Parramatta and Pittwater.

The first large group of "Chinese travellers," as they came to be derisively known, took off from Rose Hill in November 1791 – twenty men and one woman, Irish convicts off the Queen. They separated, blundered about in the bush for days, and in their starving bewilderment were easily recaptured (although three of them were so sure they had nearly reached China that they soon ran away again, and died). In time, the China myth was joined by another fancy, reported by Collins with his usual disapproval of the croppies who held it: "In addition to their natural vicious propensities, they conceived an opinion that there was a colony of white people, which had been discovered in this country, situated to the SW of the settlement, from which it was distant between three and four hundred miles." This other Shangri-la, where no work ever needed to be done, sustained some hope for a time.

In 1798 the Irish were still running away to China, as many as sixty people at a time. Since none of them had a compass (and few possessed any idea of how to use it even if they had had one), they went out armed with a magical facsimile consisting of a circle crudely sketched on paper or bark with the cardinal points but no needle.

166 In lines 2 and 3, Hughes evokes fantastic, iconic images of the Orient. These images correspond to a general impression held by

    A the author
    B the British government
    C the Chinese
    D the "Chinese travellers"

167 The lead-in about and quote from Collins in lines 14-18 suggests his view of the convicts is both

    A compassionate and paternalistic
    B bigoted and paternalistic
    C fearful and suspicious
    D bigoted and fearful

168 The overarching tone of this passage would be best described as

    A ironic and restrained
    B wildly humourous
    C politically strident
    D incredulous and angry

169 The fact that the Irish were still attempting the impossible escape to China in 1798 (lines 20-25) indicates very highly that as a group

    A they were afraid of hard work
    B they were seduced by the attractiveness of the Orient
    C they were subjected to extreme hardship in bondage
    D they were susceptible to rumors

170 It could be argued that the tale of the needle-less compass in lines 21-24 might be also be used by Hughes as a metaphor for

    A the futility of human effort
    B colonialism
    C the fight for justice
    D fear of the unknown

UNIT 38 - Stephen J. Pyne "Burning Bush"

This passage is taken from Stephen J. Pyne's *Burning Bush: A Fire History of Australia.*

THE ANCESTRAL DREAMTIME was at least partially conceived and animated by fire. As a context, fire invited contemplation, and as an object, it demanded explanation. The reverie induced by fire helped transport narrators back to the Dreamtime; staring into flame brought magicians to a trance from which they could communicate with the spirit world; the vital stories of creation and existence were almost always told or reenacted around a fire. It is too much to argue, as Bachelard has for humans in general, that fire was the originating phenomenon of mental activity, "the first phenomenon, on which the human mind reflected." But one could agree with him that the "mind in its primitive state, together with its poetry and its knowledge, had been developed in meditation before a fire." The Dreaming was likely illuminated, if not inspired, by fire.

The pervasiveness of fire in Aboriginal Dreaming reflects the pervasiveness of fire in Aboriginal life. Fire practices created a repertoire of actions and effects that could be transfigured into stories and symbols. But once in this cognitive realm humans could reassemble the pieces according to other kinds of logic. They could establish new patterns that relied on emotional or symbolic associations, without analogues in actual life; like a collage, they could alter the individual parts to make a larger truth, a new register of meanings. From this register came a cognitive universe that told the Aborigine who he was, and a moral universe that informed him how he should behave. Through its metamorphosis into a parallel mental universe, the significance of fire in Aboriginal Australia expanded far beyond its presence in the landscape.

171 What is the author's argument, in contrast with Bachelard's argument in lines 7-8?

   A fire initiated the first processes of human thought
   B fire was the only element that inspired the Dreaming
   C fire was the entire foundation of Aboriginal mythology
   D fire was a formative part of the development of the Dreaming

172 According to Bachelard's theories, what might fire symbolize for the human being?

    A hearth and the home
    B passion
    C the mind
    D life/animating force

173 The "new patterns" Pyne mentions in lines 16-17 are in some ways analogous to

    A everyday life
    B the landscape of the bush
    C dreams
    D fire

174 In the last paragraph of this passage, Pyne suggests that, through its influence on Aboriginal thought and dreaming, fire had a significant (if indirect) effect on Aboriginal

    A views on death and dying
    B social mores
    C life span
    D relationship with elders

175 Another way of stating what the author claims in lines 20-21 is that fire

    A transformed from beyond the material into a whole new realm of thinking
    B always remained a mystery to the Aborigines
    C left its mark upon the native Aboriginal landscape
    D was far more significant a concept to the Aborigines than to Westerners

UNIT 39 - Thomas Keneally "Outback"

This passage is taken from Thomas Keneally's *Outback*.

EVERY AUGUST, THE town fathers of Alice Springs celebrate a regatta in the Todd River. With the sort of surreal whimsicality which characterizes Australians in remote places, they call the event Henley-on-Todd and the whimsy consists in this: that the Todd only flows after rare heavy rains. The regatta is therefore held in the dry sand of the river bed. The organizes yearly take out insurance against rain. To have water in the Todd would spoil the regatta, would send thousands of visitors away, would bring down commercial disaster.

The yachts which compete in Henley-on-Todd have sails but no keels. Squads of brawny central Australians step into them, lift them by means of bars running athwart the vessels, and take off with them, running in unison. The running has to be in time. If those who are carrying a yacht get out of step with each other, the craft will nose-dive into the sand, the runners in the stern will be projected backside over tip through the rigging, perhaps head-first through the mainsail. Paddle races are held too – single sculls to eights. Racing shells have wheels attached and run on rails. It is all done on great heat and with preposterous energy. Because it is the best sort of joke, it is spitting in the eye of the gods who made the dry, un-European Centre. It is a case of addressing the Australian God of Weather, Hughie, and telling him to stick his bloody rain.

It is, of course, a white celebration. The Aboriginals, who have been living along dry beds since the last Ice Age, cannot be expected to get the point…Until recently, right in the centre of Alice, the dry bed of the Todd – one of the world's most ancient rivers – was peopled by Aboriginal alcoholics and their families, as well, of course, as by people in from the settlements on a temporary binge. A recent ordinance forbidding public consumption of liquor within a two-kilometre radius of Alice has moved the river-bed dwellers either north or south of town. It is an improbable life that is led there between the banks of the river. "If you had to define hell, "said a Northern Territory cop, "it would be the existence of an Aboriginal kid living with his parents in the Todd bed."

176 In lines 1-5, Keneally paints the white Australians of Alice Springs as having a heightened collective

  A sense of devoutness
  B sense of impending doom
  C sense of the absurd
  D business sense

177 In contrast with the existence of the Todd-dwelling Aboriginals, other Aboriginals' and white settlers' relationship to alcohol seems less desperate. In which line or lines do you find evidence for this statement?

   A line 28
   B lines 26-29
   C line 20
   D line 24

178 The attitude of the Northern Territory cop toward the Todd-dwelling Aborigines could be construed as

   A compassionate
   B judgmental
   C dispassionate
   D admiring

179 By juxtaposing the long description of the white settlers' celebration with the last paragraph, Keneally underscores

   A the contrast between the dryness of the bush and the water-wealth of Western Europe
   B the contrast between the life circumstances of the alcoholics and those of the average resident of Alice
   C the contrast between life circumstances of white settlers and Aboriginal bed-dwellers
   D the contrast between his own beliefs and those of the Northern Territory cop

180 The ordinance forbidding public consumption of liquor in and around Alice had the effect of

   A increasing the area population's dependence on alcohol
   B strengthening the financial circumstances of the Aboriginal population
   C displacing the alcohol-dependent population
   D popularizing Henley-on-Todd

UNIT 40 - David Malouf "Closer"

Please read this extract from David Malouf's short story 'Closer' and answer the questions which follow.

My name is Amy, but in the family I am called Ay, and my brothers, Mark and Ben, call me Rabbit. Next year, when I am ten, and can think for myself and resist the influences, I will go to school like the boys. In the meantime my grandmother teaches me. I am past long division. Uncle Charles is the eldest, the first-born. When you see him in family photographs with my mother and Uncle James and Uncle Matt, he is the blondest; his eyes have the most sparkle to them. My mother says he was always the rebel. She says his trouble is he never grew up. He lives in Sydney, which Grandpa Morpeth says is Sodom. This is the literal truth, as Aaron's rod when he threw it at Pharoah's feet did literally become a serpent and Jesus turned water into wine. The Lord destroyed Sodom and he is destroying Sydney, but with fire this time that is slow and invisible. It is burning people up but you don't see it because they burn from within. That's at the beginning. Later, they burn visibly, and the sight of the flames blistering and scorching and blackening and wasting to the bone is terrible.

Because Uncle Charles lives in Sodom we do not let him visit. If we did, we might be touched. He's one of the fools in Israel, that is what Grandpa Morpeth calls him. He has practised abominations. Three years ago he confessed this to my Grandpa and Grandma and my Uncles James and Matt, expecting them to welcome his frankness. Since then he is banished. He is as water spilled on the ground that cannot be gathered up again. So that we will not be infected by the plague he carries, Grandpa has forbidden him to come on to the land. In fact he is forbidden to come at all, though he does come at Easter and Christmas, when we see him across the home-paddock fence. He stands far back on the other side and my grandfather and grandmother and the rest of us stand on ours, on the grass slope below the house.

We live in separate houses but on the same farm, which is where my mother and Uncle James and Uncle Matt and Uncle Charles when he was young, grew up, and where my Uncles James and Matt still work.

They are big men with hands swollen and scabbed from the farm work they do, and burnt necks and faces, and feet with toenails grey from sloshing about in rubber boots in the bails. They barge about the kitchen at five o'clock in their undershorts, still half asleep, then sit waiting for Grandma to butter their toast and pour their tea. Then they go out and milk the herd, hose out the bails, drive the cows to pasture and cut and stack lucerne for winter feed–sometimes my brothers and I go with them. They are blond like Uncle Charles, but not so blond, and the hair that climbs out above their singlets, under the adam's apple, is dark. They are jokers, they like to fool about, they are always teasing. They have a wild streak but have learned to keep it in. My mother says they should marry and have wives.

181 In line 2, 'next year, when I am ten... and can think for myself and resist the influences', the tone suggests that...

    A Amy is exceptionally articulate for her age.
    B Amy is quoting from an older family member.
    C Amy is concerned about negative influences she may come under.
    D Amy is aware of the fact that she cannot yet think for herself.

182 At the end of the first paragraph, the lines 'Later, they burn visibly...the sight of the flames blistering and scorching and blackening and wasting to the bone is terrible' suggest Amy...

    A is terrified at the thought of such afflictions.
    B does not believe in these tales of horror.
    C has misunderstood the situation.
    D is fascinated by what she imagines happening.

183 Uncle Charles has been exiled from the family because...

    A he has left the family farm to live in corrupt Sydney.
    B he has committed serious crimes.
    C he has admitted being homosexual.
    D he has an infectious disease which they may catch.

184 The description, 'we see him across the home-paddock fence...' implies

   A that Charles is hurt by the family's attitude.
   B that the family miss Charles.
   C that there is distance emotionally and physically between them.
   D that Charles has never been part of the family.

185 Amy's description of her uncles in the last paragraph suggests she feels...

   A disgusted and yet fascinated by the men.
   B frightened of their teasing.
   C shy yet quietly fond of them.
   D an anxious desire to be liked by them.

186 Amy's religious beliefs are...

   A a result of indoctrination
   B strong and decided
   C unsure and born of fear
   D obsessive and unhealthy

UNIT 41 - Eve D. Fesi

The following is an excerpt of an article written by Eve D. Fesi of the Gabi Gabi tribe.

The word 'aborigine' refers to an indigenous person of any country. If it is to be used to refer to us as a specific group of people, it should be spelled with a capital 'A', i.e. 'Aborigine'. The word 'aboriginal' is an adjective used to describe something associated with aborigines, for example 'aboriginal paintings'. It should be spelled with a capital 'A' when it refers to something associated with our people. So why is the form 'Aboriginal' used, ungrammatically, as a noun when the word should be 'Aborigine'? With a few exceptions, e.g. Commonwealth and Victorian Departments of Education, you will notice governmental departments always refer to Australian Aborigines as 'Aboriginals' because they were instructed to do so. To find out the reason, we must go back to 1901.

The law at the time gave the Commonwealth power to legislate in relation to any race of people except 'aboriginal natives'. Thus, through British law and the use of the term 'aboriginal natives', we were denied an identity as a race of people. An 'opinion' was sought from government legal officers, who advised that 'aboriginal natives' should continue to be excluded from that law and that we should be known as aboriginal citizens or natives (note the small 'a'). The term 'aboriginal', meaning aboriginal native or citizen, came into use as a noun and in the case of more than one person was changed to aboriginals, meaning aboriginal natives.

Later, we demanded that Aborigine be spelled with a capital 'A', the capital 'A' was also used on Aboriginals, which still implies Aboriginal natives and a denial of our identity. The worst thing about the use of 'Aboriginals' is that it places us into the category of being a non-existent people, thus sustaining the 'legality' of the terra nullius annexation of our land. Misuse of the English language in this word reinforces the attempts to wipe out our identity and our race.

Just as we demanded capital 'A' for Aborigine, we demand Aborigine not 'Aboriginal' except in the correct place as an adjective.

187 Usage of the word 'aboriginal' is motivated by

    A political powers
    B revised legislation
    C language restrictions
    D indigenous traditions

188 What does capitalizing 'Aborigine' signify?

   A legislation against indigenous people
   B legal definition of an indigenous people
   C formal recognition of an indigenous people
   D allowance of equality among indigenous people

189 How does a lack of capitalization affect a people's identity?

   A It clarifies the existence of a group.
   B It allows equal protection under the law.
   C It diminishes their importance within a society.
   D It limits a group's ability to change legislation.

190 Refusing to capitalize 'aborigine' or 'aboriginal' is an act of

   A assertion
   B legislation
   C affirmation
   D discrimination

191 Fesi's article is an attempt to

   A seek political action
   B understand tradition
   C reject discrimination
   D formalize an identity

Modern Prose

UNIT 42 - D.J. Waldie "Holy Land: A Suburban Memoir"

This passage is taken from D.J. Waldie's *Holy Land: A Suburban Memoir*.

[Chapter] 167

AT FIRST, IT wasn't a city at all.
   The developers called it a "$250,000,000 planned community."
   According to the engineering drawings, it was 105 acres of concrete sidewalks and 133 miles of paved streets lined with 5,000 concrete light poles. These were paid for by the three developers.
   It was the service roads that paralleled the major streets, to keep traffic out of residential neighborhoods.
   According to the sales brochure, it was two coats of paint on the interior walls and wallpaper above the chair rail in the dining room.
   It was a garbage disposal in every kitchen. The sales brochure said the new suburb was "the only garbage-free city in the world."
   It also was the developers' promise of twenty elementary schools, thirty-seven playgrounds, and eighteen churches. The sales brochure said the suburb would have "churches of every denomination." The brochure listed twenty-six.
   The list of denominations is not alphabetized. Between Presbyterian and Adventist is listed Synagogue.

192 Line 2 and the repetition of the phrases "the sales brochure said" and "according to the sales brochure" (lines 7, 10, 13, 15) seem to indicate that before it was a city, Waldie's suburb was

   A a fantasy
   B a commodity
   C a community
   D a small town

193 The picture Waldie paints of his city-to-be in lines 3-5 is

   A welcoming
   B alienating
   C circuitous
   D sterile

194 In this passage's many quotes, the features of the "$250,000,000 planned community" are represented as

   A absurd
   B false
   C artificial
   D desirable

195 The title of the book, "Holy Land," could either be ironic or imply that to Waldie, his city is literally a place of

   A pilgrimage
   B artifice
   C disaster
   D deviance

196 Lines 16 and 17 could possibly imply some judgment on the part of the suburb's sales department in respect to

   A The importance of religion in the United States
   B The religious demographics of its potential population
   C The quality of religious education available to its residents
   D Relative interpretations of religious texts among its potential population

UNIT 43 - Italo Calvino "Six Memos For the Next Millennium"

This passage is taken from Italo Calvino's *Six Memos For the Next Millennium*.

WHY DO I feel the need to defend values that many people might take to be perfectly obvious? I think that my first impulse arises from a hyper-sensitivity or allergy. It seems to me that language is always used in a random, approximate, careless manner, and this distresses me unbearably. Please don't think that my reaction is the result of intolerance toward my neighbor: the worst discomfort at all comes from hearing myself speak. That's why I try to talk as little as possible. If I prefer writing, it is because I can revise each sentence until I reach the point where – if not exactly satisfied with my words – I am able at least to eliminate those reasons for dissatisfaction that I can put a finger on. Literature – and I mean the literature that matches up to these requirements – is the Promised Land in which language becomes what it really ought to be.

It sometimes seems to me that a pestilence has struck the human race in its most distinctive faculty – that is, the use of words. It is a plague afflicting language, revealing itself as a loss of cognition and immediacy, an automatism that tends to level out all expression into the most generic, anonymous, and abstract formulas, to dilute meanings, to blunt the edge of expressiveness, extinguishing the spark that shoots out from the collision of words and new circumstances.

197 Calvino's tone in this passage could be characterized, in part, as

    A ironic
    B clipped
    C conversational
    D misanthropic

198 Calvino makes great claims for Literature with a capital "L" in lines 10-12. What does he seem to be saying language "really ought to be?"

    A dilute
    B specific
    C concrete
    D adequate

199 In relation to other humans' use of language, Calvino seems to consider himself

    A superior
    B inferior
    C faulty
    D obsessive

200 According to Calvino, the distinguishing quality of humanity is our

    A faculty for language
    B ability to express emotion
    C willingness to change
    D use of language

201 The author prefers writing to speaking primarily because

    A Writing is a solitary activity, and he prefers solitude to social interaction
    B He hates the sound of his own voice and would rather be silent
    C He detests the sound of others' voices and thinks little of people in general
    D Writing allows him to approximate what he wishes to express

UNIT 44 - Keith Basso "Wisdom Sits in Places"

This passage is taken from Keith Basso's *Wisdom Sits in Places: Landscape and Language Among the Western Apache.*

AN UNFAMILIAR LANDSCAPE, like an unfamiliar language, is always   1
a little daunting, and when the two are encountered together – as they are,
commonly enough, in those out-of-the-way communities where ethnographers
tend to crop up – the combination may be downright unsettling. From the
outset, of course, neither landscape nor language can be ignored. On the   5
contrary, the shapes and colors and contours of the land, together with the
shifting sounds and cadences of native discourse, thrust themselves upon the
newcomer with a force so vivid and direct as to be virtually inescapable. Yet
for all their sensory immediacy (and there are occasions, as any ethnographer
will attest, when the sheer constancy of it grows to formidable proportions)   10
landscape and discourse seem resolutely out of reach. Although close at hand
and tangible in the extreme, each in its own way appears remote and inaccessible,
anonymous and indistinct, and somehow, implausibly, a shade less than fully
believable. And neither landscape nor discourse, as if determined to accentuate
these conflicting impressions, may seem the least bit interested in having them   15
resolved. Emphatically "there" but conspicuously lacking in accustomed forms
of order and arrangement, landscape and discourse confound the stranger's efforts
to invest them with significance, and this uncommon predicament, which produces
nothing if not uncertainty, can be keenly disconcerting.   19

202 One may infer from this passage that the author, as an ethnographer, has often been

    A an intrinsic part of the landscape
    B an alien in a new context
    C the only stranger in the setting he describes
    D at ease in the setting he describes

203 As is perhaps unusual for a scholar and a scientist, Basso opens by asserting his

    A hypothesis
    B expertise
    C discomfort
    D own personality

204 What two things are strongly linked in this passage?

    A out-of-the-way communities and ethnographers
    B out-of-the-way-communities and the senses
    C landscape and language
    D language and ethnographers

205 Lines 16-18, restated, might say that

    A Laying familiar contexts over new and unfamiliar ones will not necessarily make the new contexts understandable.
    B The ethnographer's previous studies and experiences will help to decipher new and strange situations
    C A visitor in an alien landscape is at risk of losing his identity and sense of balance
    D Landscape and language may not be individually explicable, but independent of each other they are more likely to be understood.

206 The author seems to infuse landscape and language with almost human qualities in what line or lines?

    A lines 4-5
    B line 1
    C line 11
    D lines 14-16

UNIT 45 - Soldiers Against Crime, or Police in a Community?

The passages in this section are from the article *Soldiers Against Crime, or Police in a Community?*

Passage I
One of the problems in writing about police, particularly detectives, is that most of our impressions come from literature rather than an examination of what police actually do. From Sherlock Holmes to Philip Marlowe the detective is portrayed as a character of strong moral fibre with the intellectual capacity to unravel complex clues and put the bad guy away. He is usually individualistic with a few close associates within the police department, but often at odds with the hierarchy of the police, who are seen as either corrupt or too soft and too liberal to do what the job requires.

207 This passage implies that in real life, detectives often work

    A without cooperation.
    B on mysterious cases.
    C with help from others.
    D while sitting at a desk.

Passage II
It is something of a myth that detectives solve crimes by assiduous collection of evidence. For the crimes that most concern the public — assaults, murders, rapes and robberies — it is the actions taken by the patrol police who get to the scene first that determine the outcome. They need to quickly find out what happened, identify suspects, collect physical evidence, and most importantly identify those who can give reliable testimony. Immediacy of investigation can be more important than specialist skills.

208 According to this passage, solving a violent crime depends on the quality of work done by

    A laboratory technicians.
    B the first police at the scene.
    C prosecuting lawyers.
    D thoughtful detectives.

Passage III
Detectives have a high status within departments and criminal investigation is seen as the epitome of police work. Elevation to criminal investigation work usually involves an elevation in rank and brings with it certain privileges; civilian clothes mean one is not constantly identified as a police officer. Detectives have a similar kind of freedom to journalists working on a story — they both exist by their contacts. These contacts' — informers' — names often need to be kept confidential, even from the boss, so it is frequently hard to know if they are really on the job or not.

209 This passage suggests that for a detective, working in police uniform

    A is very dangerous.
    B commands respect.
    C is a great privilege.
    D attracts attention.

210 It is implied in this passage that detectives may misuse their position by

    A inventing imaginary informants.
    B wearing casual clothing to work.
    C keeping secrets from their superiors.
    D giving information to journalists.

211 Passage III describes real-life detectives in a way that contrasts with the mention of

    A "strong moral fibre" in Passage I.
    B "intellectual capacity" in Passage I.
    C "reliable testimony" in Passage II.
    D "specialist skills" in Passage II.

UNIT 46 - Tim Winton "Dirt Music"

(from Tim Winton's *Dirt Music*)

A few miles north he anchors and goes over the side and right away he wishes he   1
hadn't bothered with the wetsuit; days like today you want to feel it barebacked. There's a
delirium in the water, something special in the way the reef morphs and throbs below. He
hangs at the surface a few moments to hyperventilate and then he kicks down through the
enfolded layers, the unseen byways of current and the changes of temperature that   5
lace the clear water. From a hole in the reef a groper slides out into the open in a blue-green
blast of light. Fox doesn't even load the spear. The big fish rolls aside to watch him. He
hovers motionless over soft corals and sponges, across hard yellow plate and rifts of
purple-blue. There's staghorn and brain coral, eels and blennies and blackarse cod and the
feelers of a hundred wary rock lobsters. The sea is thick with clicks and   10
rattles, the encrypted static of the silent world speaking. Pressure tightens his skin and
current roots through his hair. You could stay here, he thinks. On a single breath you
could live here on a God-given day like this when plankton spin before your eyes and fish
leave their redoubts in phalanxes to swim to you. The thread of heat inside him trickles
back to a thudding core. There's no discomfort now, no impulse to take another breath.   15
Way up there his boat hangs from the anchor rope like a party balloon. It looks so buoyant,
so beautiful, that he has to go back and see. He kicks up lazily. From too far and too long
down. Poisoned and happy. A distant part of him knows how close he's come to shallow
water blackout, but as he crashes through the glittering surface where his body still does the
breathing for him, the rest of him settles for simple ecstasy. He lies   20
half in the world. Tingling.

212 Winton evokes the atmosphere of an underwater world by

    A using descriptive sensory language, including sight and sound
    B using simile
    C relating the effect of the submersion on the body
    D all of the above

213 The author builds suspense in the passage by using the phrase

    A "you want to feel it barebacked" (line 2)
    B "the big fish rolls aside" (line 7)
    C "Pressure tightens his skin" (line 11)
    D "Way up there his boat hangs" (line 16)

214 Fox's reluctance to resurface shows

   A a wish to rethink his life
   B the magnetic quality of the primal
   C his death wish
   D an addiction to high risk, extreme sports

215 The core tension between body and mind in the dive is best expressed by the contradictory phrase

   A "There's a delirium" (lines 2-3)
   B "The sea is thick" (line 10)
   C "Poisoned and happy" (line 18)
   D "his body still does the breathing for him" (lines 19-20)

216 "He lies half in the world. Tingling." refers to Fox's experience of having been

   A consumed, perhaps changed, by a vastly different and beautiful world
   B almost immortal
   C half good, half evil
   D chilled from being underwater

UNIT 47 - Samuel Alexander "Space, Time, and Deity, Vol. 1"

The following are excerpts from Samuel Alexander's *Space, Time, and Deity, Vol. 1*

Passage I

"In saying that when I imagine an object I locate it somewhere in the same Space wherein I enjoy myself, I do not mean that I locate it somewhere in front of my eyes. On the contrary, I locate it in the place in Space to which it actually belongs. If it is the image of the Soudan I locate it in the south of Egypt. For the imaged Space is but perceived Space as it appears in an imaged form. All images of external objects are themselves spatial in character, and their parts have position relatively to each other. But also they have position in the whole of Space so far as we imagine the rest of Space. Now images are for the most part isolated objects, cut off more or less completely from their surroundings, and so far as this is the case the image as a whole cannot be said to have position at all. But directly we ask where the image is we begin to supply in image the rest of Space. Thus if I can remember the map and bear in mind the way I am facing, I image the Soudan more or less accurately where I know it to be, or in other words where it actually is."

Passage II

"The place of an image is its position in imaged Space, and according to the fullness of that imagination will its place be determined accurately or become so shadowy as almost to vanish. How the place in imaged Space is correlated with the place in perceived Space which is imaged in imaged Space, is discovered by experience, as for example, to take a very simple case, I recognise that the image of a person in front of me when I first look at him and then shut my eyes belongs to the same place as the percept of the same person. When the image is not the image of anything actual its place in actual Space is of course not actual either. This only means that the object imaged is not actual in the form which it assumes. It purports to have a place in Space, which is not actually filled by any such object. The Space which is imaged is still the same Space as is perceived, but it is occupied with imagined objects. Further discussion of the problems thus suggested belongs to a later part of our inquiry."

Passage III

"We have on the side of mind, flashes of light on a dim background of consciousness: and on the object side, more vivid or interesting particulars rising like peaks out of a continuous range of mountainous country. Thus rather than to say we are definite acts of mind which

take cognisance of a definite object, it is truer to say that every object we know is a
fragment from an infinite whole and every act of mind is correspondingly a fragment out of
a larger though finite mass."

4

6

217 After reading all three passages we can determine that the author:

    A Has a vast imagination.
    B Is concerned only with actual space.
    C Can imagine, clearly, the Soudan.
    D Believes that the mind is an occupant of space and that space is an occupant of the mind.

218 With consideration of passage II lines 1-2 and passage III lines 1-3 we can infer that:

    A Events that are not important to us become shadowed and vague.
    B The import of an event determines the accurate placement in mind and space.
    C Imagination is not correlated with the actual existence of objects.
    D All images in the mind are just as clear as the day they were experienced.

219 Considering Passage I lines 4-7 and Passage II lines 3-9 we can deduce that:

    A Images are part of the space that makes up portions of the mind's eye or imagination.
    B Images are clearly parts of actual space.
    C If images are not part of actual space then they do not truly exist.
    D Space is irrelevant regarding memories.

220 Considering Passage I in its entirety we can surmise that:

    A Imagined space is actual space.
    B By imagining an object or place we can make it a permanent and useful part of the space that occupies the mind.
    C If you know what a place looks like then you will know how to get there.
    D Images are not reliant upon the mind or space.

221 In passage II lines 3-9 and passage III lines 1-6 the author implies that:

   A All that we see is filed away for later comparison and used within the space of our mind.
   B Space is never really occupied it is only perceived to be.
   C All that we have accomplished, known and seen occupies the space within our minds as fragmented pieces that are the makeup of a greater mass that helps us to understand what we are yet to experience.
   D We directly determine and control that which occupies the space within our minds and the space that surrounds us.

UNIT 48 - "Government Not Rattled by Fuel Policy Attack"

Read the following article from *The Daily Telegraph* and answer the questions that follow.

"Govt not rattled by fuel policy attack" - June 03, 2008

Deputy Prime Minister Julia Gillard rejected the suggestion Labor has been rattled by a sustained attack from the opposition over the Government's petrol policy. The Opposition has been on the front foot in the past week, capitalising on Government embarrassment over a number of high-level leaks and doubts over the proposed FuelWatch scheme. Liberal leader Brendan Nelson has benefited with a jump in the polls. But Ms Gillard last night denied the Government had been rattled by the Opposition's attacks on its proposed fuel monitoring scheme.

"What has driven the Government in this period is what has driven us all along, and that's been about delivering our promises, including those important promises to help working families and individuals deal with their cost-of-living pressures," she told ABC television. Ms Gillard defended FuelWatch, saying it was about monitoring fuel prices and enabling people to identify the cheapest petrol in their vicinity.

But she sidestepped questions about whether the experience of the last week had left her worried about the Government's ability to sell the merits of its carbon trading scheme and the hike in energy prices it is likely to cause.

"I think what the Australian community said very clearly at the last election was that they understand that this nation has to grapple with the challenges of climate change. "They didn't want a Government that was in climate-change denial, they wanted to see a Government dealing with those challenges."

222 What accusation is Julia Gillard keen to deny?

    A That the government's current petrol policy is unreasonable.
    B That she is personally worried about the fuel situation.
    C That the Labour party are disconcerted by opposition to their fuel policies.
    D That the Opposition have a right to resist the spiralling fuel costs.

223 How does Julia Gillard defend her political party, and the government as a whole?

    A By changing the subject from perceived failures to previous victories.
    B By making relevant excuses for the party's policies.
    C By reminding the public of established governmental commitments.
    D By explaining the social conscience which motivates governmental decisions.

224 Which phrase best describes Gillard's attitude?

    A Defensive and elucidative.
    B Pugnacious and pessimistic.
    C Self sacrificing and changeable.
    D Discursive and perfidious.

225 How does Gillard approach the topic of energy prices?

    A She plays down the risk of increasing fuel costs.
    B She points out the necessity of changes in energy usage as a result of climate change.
    C She is quiet on specific issue of energy costs but praises the public's attitude to dealing with climate change.
    D She ignores the issue completely.

226 The key aim of this article is to…

    A educate the public about the debates surrounding the fuel crisis.
    B inform the reader of the Government's reaction to recent criticism.
    C highlight the prospect of rising fuel costs and shortages.
    D chronicle the conflict between supporters of the Government and Opposition.

227 Select the phrase which has the most similar meaning to line 4, 'The Opposition has been on the front foot in the past week'.

   A The Opposition has recently gained popularity.
   B The Opposition has been taking advantage of the situation recently.
   C The Opposition is always a step ahead.
   D The Opposition appears to know what is going to happen before it happens.

Conceptual Thinking

UNIT 49 - Signal Flares

In order to discover the properties of various mixtures of Strontium Nitrate, Potassium Nitrate and Wood Meal (to gather data necessary for manufacturing signal flares), several different mixtures were tested. The triangle diagram below represents graphically the results of this experimental series.

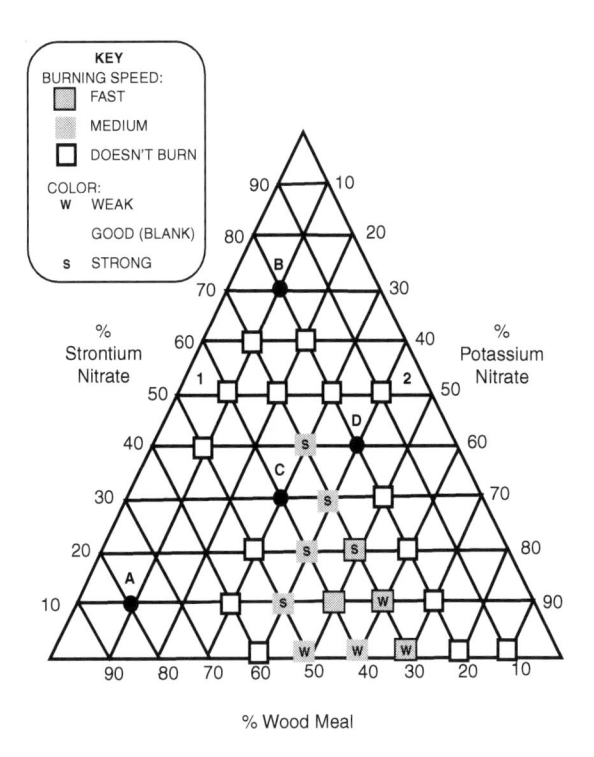

Triangle diagrams are read as percentage of each ingredient. The point labeled A in the diagram shows where a mixture of 80% Wood Meal, 10% Strontium Nitrate and 10% Potassium Nitrate would be recorded.

Each mixture was ignited to determine the burn rate and quality of perceived color. The symbols appearing on the graph are taken directly from the key and show the general results for any particular mixture. Symbols for burn rate and color are combined for each mixture recorded. Mixtures were prepared by varying quantities at steps of 10% by weight.

228 What percentages of each chemical does point B indicate?

    A Wood Meal, 20%; Strontium Nitrate, 80%
    B Strontium Nitrate, 70%; Potassium Nitrate, 30%
    C Strontium Nitrate, 70%; Wood Meal, 20%; Potassium Nitrate, 10%
    D Potassium Nitrate, 10%; Wood Meal, 90%

229 The line of open boxes running horizontally across the graph between the numbers 1 and 2 allow us to conclude which of the following?

    A Mixtures containing more than 50% Potassium Nitrate probably won't burn.
    B Mixtures containing more than 50% Strontium Nitrate probably won't burn.
    C Mixtures containing less than 50% Potassium Nitrate probably won't burn.
    D A mixture consisting of 50% Strontium Nitrate and 50% Potassium Nitrate doesn't burn.

230 The point labeled C in the diagram (if tested and recorded) is least likely to contain the symbol for:

    A Fast burning, weak color.
    B Moderate burning, strong color.
    C Moderate burning, weak color.
    D Doesn't burn

231 The point in the graph labeled D represents an experiment that wasn't recorded because the measurements were incorrect (twice as much Potassium Nitrate was weighed out than what was called for). What type of square is most likely to appear there?

    A An empty white square.
    B A shaded square with a black border.
    C A shaded square with a W in it.
    D A shaded square with a black border and an S.

232 For stability reasons, it is deemed necessary to add 10% of an inert diluent to the formulations. This stabilizer will not change the burning or color characteristics of a mixture, as long as the other ingredients remain in the same relative concentration. If it is desirable to use the existing graph, what changes would have to be made?

    A All squares would have to be shifted up one line.
    B All squares would have to be shifted down one line.
    C All numbers at the edges of the diagram have to be multiplied by 0.9.
    D There is no method that avoids repeating the experiments.

UNIT 50 - Drug Testing

A false positive result in drug testing means a test showed drug metabolites present when in fact there were none. A false negative shows no drug metabolites present when in fact there are. Background rate refers to the assumed actual drug usage rate for a given population overall.

The Brazzo company has decided to institute a drug testing program for all potential new hires. Because drug testing can be an expensive endeavor with possible legal consequences, you are asked to evaluate several possible methods.

Gotcha is a urine test strip that advertises a 5% false positive rate and a 10% false negative rate. DrugsBegone is a urine testing product that claims a 2% false positive rate and 15% false negative. Catch-It also tests urine and has a 6% false positive rate and 12% false negative.

For all of the following questions, assume that no legitimately prescribed drugs are being taken by any of the people tested. Any drug use, by this standard, is illegal. Also assume that each test uses a different detection mechanism, so that erroneous results on one test do not influence the pattern of results from a different test.

In no series of tests are all applicants either drug users or not drug users. There will always exist some mixture.

233 What order would you rank the tests (best to worst) if catching the maximum number of drug users was the primary concern of Brazzo's HR department?

    A Gotcha, DrugsBegone, Catch-It
    B DrugsBegone, Gotcha, Catch-It
    C Gotcha, Catch-It, DrugsBegone
    D Catch-It, Gotcha, DrugsBegone

234 The Legal Department at Brazzo informs you that because of possible lawsuits arising from drug testing procedures, they would like you to use a testing method that decreases the number of false positives. If Gotcha is used first, and then everyone who tests positive is then retested with DrugsBegone, what will the final overall false positive (fp) and false negative (fn) rates be?

A fp = 0.1% and fn = 23.5%
B fp = 0.1% and fn = 25%
C fp = 0.1% and fn = 1.5%
D fp > 0.1% and fn > 1.5%

235 The background rate for drug use in the demographic you are hiring from (young, college educated, professionals) is 10%. If you use Gotcha alone to test this population, what are the chances that a person who tests positive for drug use is actually a drug user? (You may round your answer up or down to choose the closest percentage.)

A 90%
B 85%
C 75%
D 67%

236 How would the chances of a positive result being correct change if you retested all positive results from the Gotcha results above (testing just the people who tested positive for drug use) with Catch-It? (Use your results from question 4 if you need to.)

A Accuracy will improve up to 99% or greater in the second group.
B There will still be a 2% chance of a false positive in the second group.
C Overall accuracy will remain the same using two tests.
D Overall accuracy will decrease using two tests.

237 A combination of testing is suggested that will use one of the three urine test strips for initial screening and anyone who tests positive will have the opportunity to test again. The second test will be through GCMS (gas chromatography/mass spectroscopy) which has a false positive rate and false negative rate very close to zero. Which of the three tests would be best to pre-screen candidates to minimize the number of drug users offered a job?

A Gotcha
B DrugsBegone
C Catch-It
D Any of them will do since GCMS is so accurate.

238 The upper management at Brazzo decides to test all 1000 of their current employees with DrugsBegone. The results are 186 positive and 814 negative. Based on this, what is the estimated background rate for drug use in this group?

A 20%
B 18.6%
C 15%
D Cannot be determined without GCMS.

UNIT 51 - Dog Coat Colour

Long before DNA was discovered and described, dog breeders and others understood the concept of inherited traits and genes. A gene was simply the unit of some quality passed from parents to offspring. Basic husbandry included the practice of selecting breeding pairs based on observed characteristics with the expectation of increasing the likelihood of those same characteristics appearing in offspring.

It is now understood that genes come in pairs (one copy from the mother and one from the father) and that genes can come in more than one variety- called alleles. A dominant allele is one that will produce an observable effect in offspring, even if it is only one of the pair of inherited genes. Dominance is shown in abbreviated form as a capital letter.

A recessive allele is the form of the gene that will only show up if both of the copies (one from the mother and one from the father) are recessive. Recessive alleles are shown as small letters.

This information can be summarized in a punnit square, which is a diagram showing all the possible combinations of parental genes and the resulting genotype of the offspring. Fig 1 shows a punnit square for two dogs and the genes for black coats.

	B	b
B	BB	Bb
b	Bb	bb

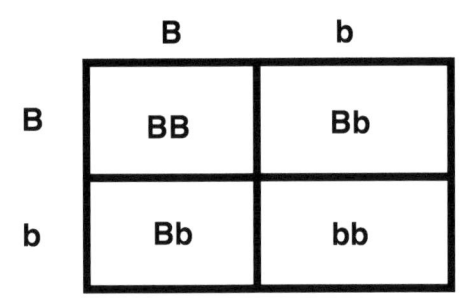

Fig. 1 Punnit Square

In the figure, the parents' genotypes are shown to the left and across the top. So, in this example, each parent carries the genotype Bb. The predicted outcome for their offspring is shown in the main four squares as BB, Bb, Bb and bb. Of these, since B is dominant and leads to a black coat color, three out of four will be black and the fourth (on average) will be recessive (bb) and be brown. In Labrador Retrievers, a brown (or chocolate) color is a recessive trait.

239 After several matings and litters, only black puppies are produced from a particular pair of dogs. Which of the following sets of genomes for the mated pair best fit this result?

A [BB, Bb] or [Bb,BB]
B [BB, Bb] or [Bb, BB] or [BB,BB]
C [BB,BB] only
D [BB,bb] or [Bb,BB] or [BB,BB]

240 An unknown male has impregnated a female black Labrador. If the subsequent litter of 9 puppies has 4 chocolates in it and 5 black dogs, which is the most likely genome for the male?

A bb
B BB
C Bb
D Either Bb or bb

Another gene if present as a recessive pair blocks the expression of dark coat color in any combination of B or b. This is referred to as the E gene.

Dogs who are ee will have a straw-colored coat and in Labradors, this is called 'yellow'. Inheritance of either allele of E is independent of B. That is, whatever combination of B genes are present has no effect on whether dominant E or recessive e is passed on to offspring.

241 A pair of black Labradors consistently has litters of only black puppies. A breeder selects dogs from one such litter and mates them together. The resulting litter of 8 from these siblings has 5 black dogs, 1 chocolate dog and 2 yellow dogs. What is the likely genome for the original pair (the grandparents of the final litter) ?

A [BBEe, BbEE] or [BBEE, BbEe]
B [BBEe, BBEE]
C [BbEE, Bb EE] or [BbEe, BbEE]
D [BbEe, BBEe] or [BBEE, BbEe]

242 If a chocolate Labrador with no recessive alleles for E is bred with a yellow Labrador, what are the chances that they will only produce black offspring?

    A 1 : 16
    B 1 : 8
    C 1 : 4
    D zero

243 A pair of Labradors are known to have BbEE and BbEe in their genomes. If they are mated and have a litter of 5 puppies, what is the approximate probability that all 5 will be black?

    A Less than 10%
    B 20%
    C 24%
    D 75%

UNIT 52 - Map Reading

Topographic Maps

Map makers have developed a system to represent three dimensional information on a two dimensional map. This is done by showing elevation on the map as contour lines and by showing spot elevations for various features.

A contour in this use means a line of equal elevation above sea level, and is given for every fifth contour line, which is drawn as a solid line (other lines appear broken in these examples). The contour interval is the vertical distance between adjacent lines. Figure 1 is an example of a topographic map with these features.

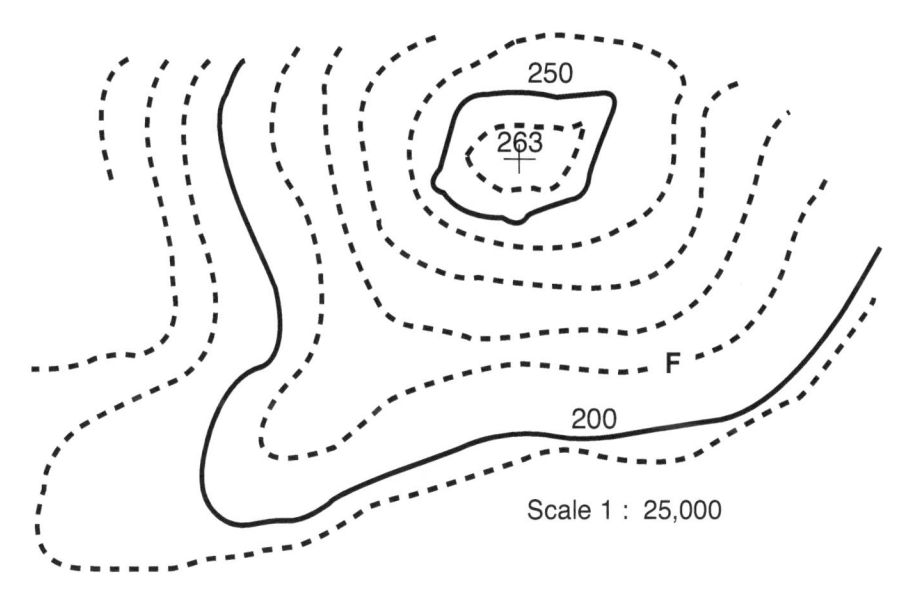

Fig. 1

Figure 1 shows a hilltop with a spot elevation of 263 meters marked. The contour interval for this map is 10 m. Point F is on an unlabeled contour line, but by interpolation, the line must be 210 m. By convention, any point not on a contour line is considered to be at an elevation half-way between the elevations on either side.

Fig. 2

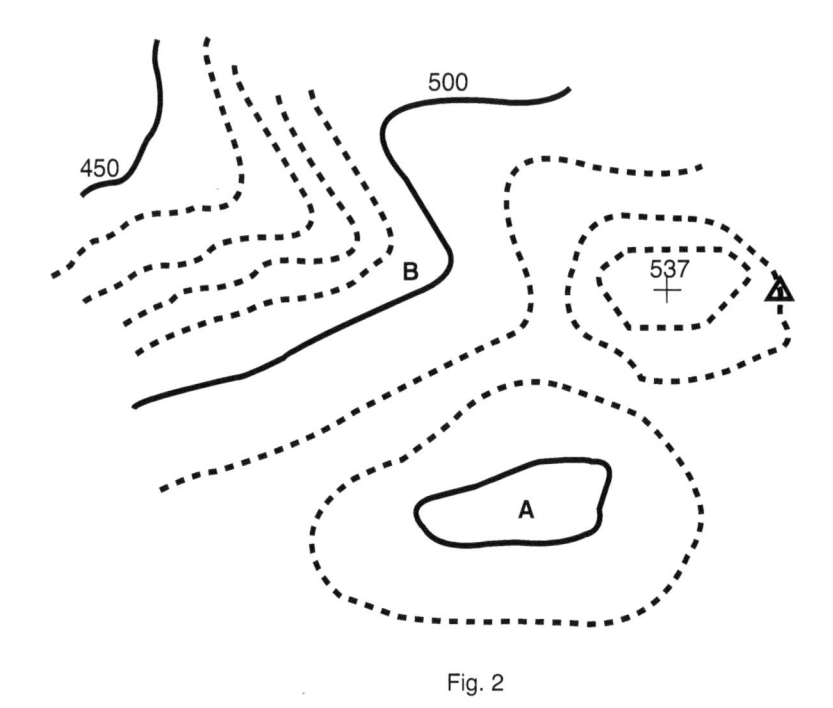

Other definitions:

Map Distance is a measurement on a map between two points. It doesn't take into consideration that a map is an extremely foreshortened representation. Map distances can never be greater than the dimensions of the actual map being used.

Ground Distance is the distance horizontally that the map distance represents. It doesn't take into consideration slope or elevation.

Linear Distance is the actual distance one would measure on the ground between points on a map. It takes into consideration the differences in elevation between two points. If two places on a map are at the same elevation and there are no significant topographic features (hills, valleys, etc.) between them, then linear and ground distance will be the same.
Scale is the relationship between map distance and ground distance. It is usually expressed as a ratio, such as-- 1:50,000. This means that 1 inch on the physical map represents a distance of 50,000 inches on the ground.

244 Point F in figure 1 is on a contour line. If the map distance between point F and the hilltop (with the listed spot elevation) is 2 cm, what is the linear distance between these two places?

A 459 m
B 500 m
C 503 m
D 523 m

245 Refer to figure 2. Travel from point A on this map to the spot elevation marked 537 would entail which of the following?

A Generally traveling uphill.
B Generally traveling downhill.
C First going uphill at least 10 m and then generally downhill.
D First going downhill at least 10 m and then generally uphill.

246 Neither point A nor point B is on a contour line. What is the difference in elevation between point A and point B?

A At most, 35 meters.
B At most, 10 meters.
C At most, 5 meters.
D They are at the same elevation.

247 Point B, the spot elevation and the triangle shown on the right of the map are aligned. If the triangle indicates a tower with a light on top, how high would the tower have to be so that the light is directly visible from point B? (The ground distance between B and the hilltop is 100 m and the ground distance between the hilltop and the tower base is 50 m.)

A 25 m
B 38 m
C 41 m
D at least 50 m

248 One key use for a topographical map is determining percent slope or grade. This is the vertical rise divided by the horizontal (ground distance) traveled expressed as a percentage. If a vehicle travels 100 meters and the elevation increases 50 meters, the grade would be 50%.

Referring to figure 2, if the map distance and scale are unknown between point B and the hilltop labeled 537 m, what is the minimum ground distance required to drive a vehicle from B to the hilltop without exceeding a 5% grade?

A Not enough information given.
B 270 m
C 430 m
D 860 m

UNIT 53 - Memory Access

Memory and Data Storage

A bit (from binary digit) can have one of two discrete states, expressed as 0 or 1. A byte consists of eight bits and can take on values from 00000000 up to 11111111, allowing for 256 different states. A word is 16 bits, or two bytes.

Memory locations are addressable areas of physical memory in a data storage system, and in the examples that follow, each location contains one word. The address of a location is written in hexadecimal format. Hexadecimal means base 16, and the digits for 10 = A, 11 = B, 12 = C, 13 = D, 14= E and 15 = F. When it isn't clear which base (2 for binary, 10 for decimal or 16 for hexadecimal) is being used a lowercase letter (b, d or h) will precede the number.

A block of addressable memory is made up of words that are referenced one to one by hexadecimal addresses in the form h0000 up to hFFFF. In these examples, the higher addresses, from hFF00 to hFFFF are reserved for non-data purposes.

(Kb refers to Kilo bytes, Mb to Mega bytes.)

249   How much memory is available to hold data?

    A   about 65 Kb
    B   about .5 Mb
    C   about 260 Kb
    D   about 130 Kb

The reserved memory locations are used to hold addresses to other memory locations and program instructions. This is possible because one word of 16 bits is equivalent to a 4 digit hexadecimal address. This arrangement is context dependent-- bits in one area of memory are interpreted as data, and bits in another area of memory are interpreted as addresses or instructions.

The location hFFFF is used to hold the current pointer. The current pointer is the address in memory where data is going to be read from next.

For example, if the value in memory location hFFFF is hA045, then the pointer is pointing to address hA045, and whatever data is in that location will be read when the pointer is referenced.

The put command takes the value at any address and copies it to another location, overwriting whatever is there. put hA23B :: hFFFF would put the value found at hA23B into hFFFF. This would result in the pointer being moved to point to whatever value was originally at memory location hA23B.

250 What would the following sequence of put commands accomplish?
put hFFFF :: h1234 ; put hEA34 :: hFFFF ; put h1234 :: hFFFF

    A The pointer will read h1234 next.
    B The value at h1234 might have changed, but not hFFFF.
    C hEA34 and h1234 will have the same value.
    D The start and end states will be the same for this sequence.

In this model, data is entered (input) into one address at a time. After each entry the pointer is increased so that the next higher memory location will hold the next item of data. Data is read (output) by decreasing the pointer by one after each data item is read. This architecture is called First In-Last Out, or FILO, because the first data item input will be the last one read. Other data structures use FIFO (first in, first out) by either manipulating the data or how the pointer moves.

251 In our model, what will the following sequence accomplish?
Input 10 data items ; read these and input them to another area of memory; read this new area of memory; output the data.

    A It will output the data in FIFO order
    B It will create two identical data lists.
    C It will randomly mix the 10 items.
    D It will move the pointer higher by h20.

252 What would the following sequence do if the data items input are: b11, b100, b101, b111 and b1000 and the value at hAB25 is h00A5?

put hAB25 :: hFFFF ; {input data} ; put h00A8 :: hFFFF ; {input data}

A b1000 will be in memory location h000B
B b11 will be in memory location h00A8
C hAB28 will have the value b111
D hFFFF will point to h0013

UNIT 54 - Plant Growth

Plant Nutrients

The major elements utilized in plant growth are Carbon (C), Nitrogen (N), Potassium (K), Hydrogen (H), Oxygen (O) and Phosphorus (P). Of these, the atmosphere and available water provide C, H, and O. The others are absorbed from the soil by most plants. Although these nutrients are used by the plant in many ways, they can be categorized as structural or functional. Structural would include cell walls, DNA and material that is largely stable- once made, structural components remain static. Functional components are made by the plant as needed and may vary over time based on different needs and environmental conditions. Functional would include enzymes and salts the plants use to maintain water balance.

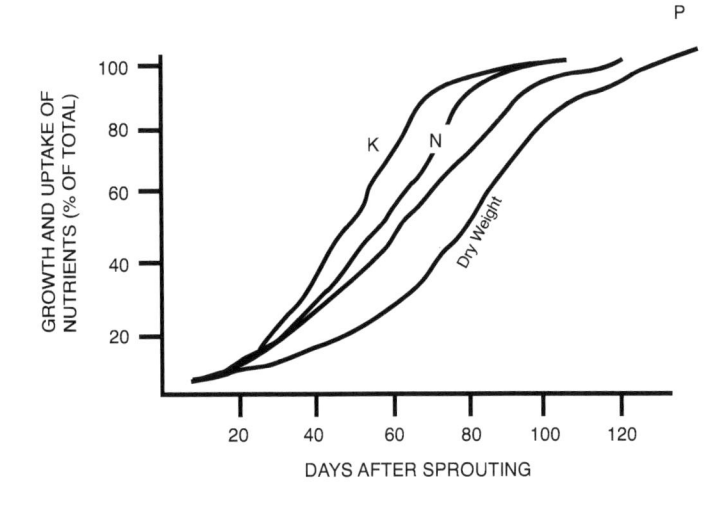

Figure 1

Figure one shows the cumulative percentage of absorbed nutrients for the growth of sorghum. Dry weight in this graph is determined by evaporating as much water as possible from the plant.

253 Which of the following does the graph imply?

    A Sorghum needs more Nitrogen than Phosphorus.
    B Potassium is the largest requirement for Sorghum (of the nutrients shown).
    C Water absorption occurs most in the last half of the growth cycle.
    D Potassium is probably a functional component.

254 The relative weight percentages of major nutrients in this plant when fully grown are listed below.

C, 45%
O, 45%
H, 6%
N, 1.5%
K, 1%
P, 0.2%

If C, O and H were combined and drawn as a single line in figure one, how would this line appear?

A To the left of Dry Weight and parallel at all points with Phosphorus.
B To the right of Dry Weight and parallel at all points with Dry Weight.
C To the left of Dry Weight and parallel at all points to Nitrogen.
D The graph wouldn't change.

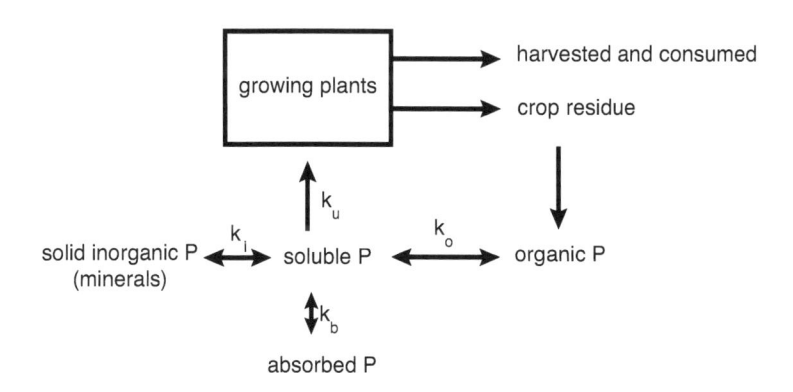

Figure 2 Phosphorus cycle

Figure 2 shows the general movements of Phosphorus during plant growth. The k's shown are rates of transfer. These are affected by factors such as soil pH, soil type (loam, clay, sand) and the amount of available water.

For instance, ki (the rate at which P from mineral sources moves to and from the soil solution) is markedly influenced by soil pH with a maximum between 6.5 and 7. This same factor (pH) also influences kb (bound or adsorbed P), and increases it when sufficient water is available. Ku and ko are not affected by a change in pH.

The amount of phosphate ions available for plant use is usually under 1 Kg/hectacre (one hectacre = 2.47 acres) while crops may require 20 to 30 lbs/acre(1 Kg = 2.2lbs) for proper growth. This means that P (as the phosphate) in the soil solution must be replenished many times during plant growth.

255 If the available phosphate per hectacre is 1 Kg and this is replenished (from ki, kb and ko) at an average rate of 1Kg/hectacre per week, how much additional phosphate from fertilizer would be required for a crop that needed 25 lb/acre over a 140 day growth period? (Assume constant uptake over the entire growth period.)

  A 15 lb/acre
  B 7.4lb/acre
  C 6.3lb/acre
  D No additional fertilizer is required.

256 Using Fig. 1 and the data from question 3, when would be the latest the fertilizer could be applied so that the crop didn't become deficient in P?

  A 2 week
  B 3 weeks
  C 4 weeks
  D 5 weeks

257 Adding lime to the soil (which started at pH 6) to raise the pH would do all of the following except what?

  A Increase the time until fertilizer was needed.
  B Increase ki and kb.
  C Shift the P curve in figure 1 to the right.
  D Reduce the amount of fertilizer needed.

UNIT 55 - Voting Systems

Simple majority, or plurality voting, is a common method used in parliamentary procedure and elections to decide issues and elect one candidate from a field of opponents. Essentially, a poll is taken of the electorate and whichever candidate or course of action receives the most votes is declared the winner.

Consider the following election, with the votes distributed as shown:
Candidate A; 45%
Candidate B; 40%
Candidate C; 10%
Candidate D; 5%

In a plurality vote, A would win with a 45% majority. This result might be satisfactory, but it suffers from some consequences. The first is that the majority of the voters do not support A, only 45% do. The second consequence is that the plurality method is vulnerable to strategic voting.

If the supporters of C knew in advance (perhaps through polling) that A was likely to win, they could vote for B instead of C and make B the winner. Strategic voting in this example allows a very small fraction (10%) of voters to control the outcome.

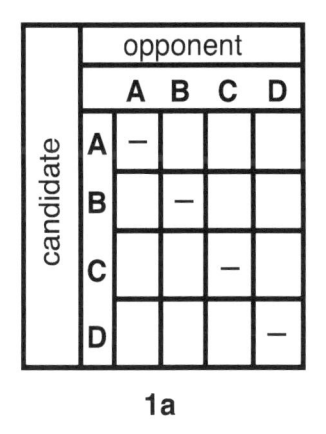

1a

	\multicolumn{4}{c}{opponent}
candidate	A	B	C	D
A	—			
B		—		
C			—	
D				—

1b

	\multicolumn{4}{c}{opponent}
candidate	A	B	C	D
A	—	1	1	1
B	0	—	0	1
C	0	1	—	1
D	0	0	0	—

Diagram 1: Condorcet Ballot

Because of these factors, other voting methods have been suggested. The Condorcet method uses ranked preferences instead of a simple majority to determine the winner. In practice, voters rate each candidate from first to last according to who they prefer most to least.

Candidates are then matched pairwise in a plurality fashion and then the totals are summed to get an overall winner.

Practically, voters are asked to fill out a ballot like that in diagram 1a, ranking each candidate one at a time against every other candidate. Ballots are filled in by rows, comparing each candidate one on one against each opponent- entering a 1 if the candidate is preferred over that particular opponent and a 0 if not.

A voter who prefers the candidates in the order of A, C, B, D would fill in the ballot as shown in diagram 1b.

258 How would a Condorcet ballot appear for a voter with the preferences B, C, A, D?

A - 1 1 0	B - 0 0 1	C - 0 0 1	D - 1 1 0
0 - 0 0	1 - 1 1	1 - 1 1	0 - 0 0
0 1 - 0	1 0 - 1	0 1 - 0	1 0 - 1
1 1 1 -	0 0 0 -	0 0 0 -	1 1 1 -

To determine the winner in a Condorcet election all the ballots are summed at each square and the summed ballot is read. If one candidate is preferred over all others, that is the Condorcet winner. An example of a summed matrix for an election with 3 voters and 4 candidates is shown in diagram 2.

	opponent				
		A	B	C	D
candidate	A	—	0	0	1
	B	3	—	3	2
	C	3	0	—	2
	D	2	1	1	—

Diagram 2

To find the winner in this example, compare each candidate with each opponent as if they were the only two candidates in an imaginary election. Comparing A to C, A received 0 votes against C (when A is the candidate- third box, top row) and C receives 3 votes when C is the candidate and A is the opponent (third row, first column). So, pairwise, C beats A.

259 Using the summed ballot shown in diagram 2, what is the overall preference order in this election?

A B, C, D, A
B B, D, C, A
C B, D & C tied, A
D C, B, D, A

260 A poll shows that voters in an election prefer candidates with the following rankings. Under the Condorcet voting method, who would win the election?

45% A, C, B, D
40% B, C, D, A
10% C, D, B, A
5%   D, B, A, C

A A
B B
C C
D no clear winner

261 Ties or unclear results can arise in most voting methods. For the Condorcet method, one way to solve this problem is to take the total number of votes in a row (on the summed ballot) and use the higher total to determine a winner when pairwise comparisons do not yield a winner.

Using this additional method on the data from question 3, what will the final ranking be for the election?

A D, A, B, C
B A, C, B, D
C C, B, D, A
D no clear preference

262 Although largely resistant to strategic voting, the Condorcet method can be influenced by burying. Burying is when people vote their first choice first, but then, no matter what their actual preference is, rank some particular candidate last; in essence, burying that candidate. If candidate B is buried in this way, what will the new ranking be for this election?

A C, D, B, A
B A, C, D, B
C C, D, A, B
D A, D, B, C

Section II Essay Topics

Creativity

The creation of something new is not accomplished by the intellect but by the play instinct acting from inner necessity. The creative mind plays with the objects it loves.

Carl Jung (1875 - 1961)

When Alexander the Great visited Diogenes and asked whether he could do anything for the famed teacher, Diogenes replied: 'Only stand out of my light.' Perhaps some day we shall know how to heighten creativity. Until then, one of the best things we can do for creative men and women is to stand out of their light.

John W. Gardner (1912 -)

The secret to creativity is knowing how to hide your sources.

Albert Einstein (1879 - 1955)

Every time we say, "Let there be!" in any form, something happens.

Stella Terrill Mann

Creativity can solve almost any problem. The creative act, the defeat of habit by originality, overcomes everything.

George Lois

Defeat

Victory attained by violence is tantamount to a defeat, for it is momentary.

Mahatma Gandhi (1869 - 1948), *'Satyagraha Leaflet No. 13,' May 3, 1919*

You can take from every experience what it has to offer you. And you cannot be defeated if you just keep taking one breath followed by another.

Oprah Winfrey (1954 -), *O Magazine, What I Know For Sure, January 2004*

Far better it is to dare mighty things, to win glorious triumphs even though checkered by failure, than to rank with those poor spirits who neither enjoy nor suffer much because they live in the gray twilight that knows neither victory nor defeat.

Theodore Roosevelt (1858 - 1919)

Be careful that victories do not carry the seed of future defeats.

Ralph W. Sockman

Victorious warriors win first and then go to war, while defeated warriors go to war first and then seek to win.

Sun-Tzu (~400 BC), *The Art of War. Strategic Assessments*

Immortality

I have Immortal longings in me.

        William Shakespeare (1564 - 1616), *"Antony and Cleopatra", Act 5 scene 2*

The soul of man is immortal and imperishable.

        Plato (427 BC - 347 BC), *The Republic*

Millions long for immortality who don't know what to do with themselves on a rainy Sunday afternoon.

        Susan Ertz, *Anger in the Sky*

Ten thousand fools proclaim themselves into obscurity, while one wise man forgets himself into immortality.

        Martin Luther King Jr. (1929 - 1968)

I don't want to achieve immortality through my work... I want to achieve it through not dying.

        Woody Allen (1935 -)

Opportunity

Trouble is only opportunity in work clothes.

Henry J. Kaiser (1882 - 1967)

Small opportunities are often the beginning of great enterprises.

Demosthenes (384 BC - 322 BC)

The Chinese use two brush strokes to write the word 'crisis.' One brush stroke stands for danger; the other for opportunity. In a crisis, be aware of the danger - but recognize the opportunity.

Richard M. Nixon (1913 - 1994)

While we stop to think, we often miss our opportunity.

Publilius Syrus (~100 BC), *Maxims*

Opportunity is missed by most people because it is dressed in overalls and looks like work.

Thomas A. Edison (1847 - 1931)

Patriotism

It is not unseemly for a man to die fighting in defense of his country.

Homer (800 BC - 700 BC), *The Iliad*

You're not to be so blind with patriotism that you can't face reality. Wrong is wrong, no matter who does it or says it.

Malcolm X (1925 - 1965)

And so, my fellow Americans: ask not what your country can do for you - ask what you can do for your country. My fellow citizens of the world: ask not what America will do for you, but what together we can do for the freedom of man.

John F. Kennedy (1917 - 1963), *Inaugural address, January 20, 1961*

You'll never have a quiet world till you knock the patriotism out of the human race.

George Bernard Shaw (1856 - 1950), *"Misalliance"*

Patriotism is often an arbitrary veneration of real estate above principles.
When I am abroad, I always make it a rule never to criticize or attack the government of my own country. I make up for lost time when I come home.

Sir Winston Churchill (1874 - 1965)

Maturity

By the time I'd grown up, I naturally supposed that I'd be grown up.

Eve Babitz

The purpose of life is to fight maturity.

Dick Werthimer

What I look forward to is continued immaturity followed by death.

Dave Barry (1947 -)

To be mature means to face, and not evade, every fresh crisis that comes.

Fritz Kunkel

There's no point in being grown up if you can't be childish sometimes.

Doctor Who

Money

Lack of money is the root of all evil.

George Bernard Shaw (1856 - 1950)

Annual income twenty pounds, annual expenditure nineteen six, result happiness. Annual income twenty pounds, annual expenditure twenty pound ought and six, result misery.

Charles Dickens (1812 - 1870), *David Copperfield, 1849*

The rich are the scum of the earth in every country.

G. K. Chesterton (1874 - 1936), *Flying Inn (1914)*

Money was never a big motivation for me, except as a way to keep score. The real excitement is playing the game.

Donald Trump (1946 -), *"Trump: Art of the Deal"*

Who is rich? He that is content. Who is that? Nobody.

Benjamin Franklin (1706 - 1790)

Risk

If you don't risk anything you risk even more.

Erica Jong

Great deeds are usually wrought at great risks.

Herodotus (484 BC - 430 BC), *The Histories of Herodotus*

There are risks and costs to a program of action. But they are far less than the long-range risks and costs of comfortable inaction.

John F. Kennedy (1917 - 1963)

In order for people to be happy, sometimes they have to take risks. It's true these risks can put them in danger of being hurt.

Meg Cabot, *The Boy Next Door*, 2002

It seems to me that people have vast potential. Most people can do extraordinary things if they have the confidence or take the risks. Yet most people don't. They sit in front of the telly and treat life as if it goes on forever.

Philip Adams

War

What difference does it make to the dead, the orphans and the homeless, whether the mad destruction is wrought under the name of totalitarianism or the holy name of liberty or democracy?

Mahatma Gandhi (1869 - 1948), *"Non-Violence in Peace and War"*

You cannot simultaneously prevent and prepare for war.

Albert Einstein (1879 - 1955), *(attributed)*

War may sometimes be a necessary evil. But no matter how necessary, it is always an evil, never a good. We will not learn how to live together in peace by killing each other's children.

Jimmy Carter (1924 -)

Politics is war without bloodshed while war is politics with bloodshed.

Mao Tse-Tung (1893 - 1976)

Never, never, never believe any war will be smooth and easy, or that anyone who embarks on the strange voyage can measure the tides and hurricanes he will encounter. The statesman who yields to war fever must realize that once the signal is given, he is no longer the master of policy but the slave of unforeseeable and uncontrollable events.

Sir Winston Churchill (1874 - 1965)

Temptation

Good habits result from resisting temptation.

Ancient Proverb

I never resist temptation because I have found that things that are bad for me do not tempt me.

George Bernard Shaw (1856 - 1950), *The Apple Cart (1930)*

I generally avoid temptation unless I can't resist it.

Mae West (1892 - 1980)

There are several good protections against temptations, but the surest is cowardice.

Mark Twain (1835 - 1910), *Following the Equator (1897)*

The only way to get rid of a temptation is to yield to it. Resist it, and your soul grows sick with longing for the things it has forbidden to itself.

Oscar Wilde (1854 - 1900), *The Picture of Dorian Gray, 1891*

Worked Solutions

1   Answer B

The clue is in the image of 'serpents of smoke trailed themselves for ever and ever' depicting Coketown as a hellish place where there is no relief from the industrial fallout, just as there is, presumably, no relief from the 'fire and brimstone' of hell. Coketown is not 'unnatural', in the sense that unchecked pollution is a natural negative result of intense industrialization. C and D are close answers.

2   Answer B

In this passage, Dickens builds up, by the accumulation of details, an endless picture of the suffocating effects of endless pollution endured by the township. This is a critique of its market-attuned economy. There seems to be some malaise -'melancholy madness'- but this is only one detail. No criticism of proprietors have been made yet. There is a mention of consumers 'saleable in the dearest' but B presents what Dickens attempts to do overall.

3   Answer D

One gathers from the passage that the very basics of existence suffice. To go beyond that is to be frivolous and extravagant.

4   Answer B

It is true that everything has to be 'facts, facts, facts' and no imagination is allowed to exist.

5   Answer A

Dickens' concern is with the dreadful routine of the workers as one can gather from the end of paragraph two.

6   Answer B

There is a stand-off by the workers though they did not go on strike in the first place but were dismissed. It was wholesale unfair dismissal. Now that they are dismissed, they will not return to work on point of the paycut. It was wholesale unfair dismissal but the overall problem as voiced by Will is the exploitation by the owners of capital.

7   Answer D

The character, Pluto is not on the same level as Will - he is not a foil and is not present to create tension. He is an audience for Will but his function is to create narrative flow – the story goes on by his asking Will questions.

8   Answer B

The candidate has to understand the meaning of the term 'symbolic violence' within the context of the passage. In this case, A, C and D are acts of 'symbolic violence'.

9   Answer A

The mill workers did not ask for this as a condition. The other three are the conditions to return to work

10   Answer B

This story can be said to be told from a Marxist conflict perspective and the defining characteristic of a society from such a perspective is economic inequality. So the candidate has to interpret it from this framework.

11   Answer A

The author begins the narrative like someone is telling a story during a conversation. It is not a nostalgic passage as there is no tone of longing for a faded past. It does not have a tone of gossip as the person is only recounting. The word 'gravity' is too severe. The first few words are normally used in many conversations about how the present circumstances are an outcome of past actions.

12 Answer **A**

Social status includes money, privilege and class and often, honour. Social status was eminently sought after in Jane Austen's time and was a predominant value. In answering this question, consider Miss Frances' choice of marriage partner.

13 Answer **B**

In the social circles of the time gossip played a role in the approval or disapproval of relationships and events. It played the function of social control. It was, of course, intrusive and had the element of envy to a great extent. The other distractors are placed there as characteristics of gossip.

14 Answer **D**

As you read you will gather that social status of the male is important. Class ('the rank of a baronet's lady') and money is mentioned several times. The only element not mentioned is love – in fact, Miss Ward 'found herself obliged to be attached' to Rev. Norris.

15 Answer **C**

Social conventions, in particular that of marriage, shape women's lives. So it is essential to follow the dictate of social conventions. Therefore Miss Ward was obliged to marry someone appropriate who happened on the scene, having no opportunity equal to her sister's.

16 Answer **A**

This phrase follows the logic of 'to disoblige her family' (who no longer have to support her) Her choice of partner made her an outcast and all relationships with her family were severed.

17 Answer **A**

He knows his obligations – and fulfills them. The answers to eliminate is thus B, C and D.

18   Answer B

This choice covers A, C and D

19   Answer D

The opening uses prediction (the impending death of the character), shock tactics (the character seemed stunned by the news), and then one wonders about the nature of his 'profession'.

20   Answer A

This question expects the candidate to realise the irony of the situation – a man who has a close knowledge of death and dying, seem so shocked at his own. It is like a denial of his own mortality.

21   Answer B

There is no implication that the character is imaginative or religious (he may be a man of religion) nor frightened. The phrase describing him is 'little troubled by passion' and the word 'cold'.

22   Answer C

A 'good' death in the sense that it is quiet, peaceful and comes upon one unbeknownst. The other options can be eliminated.

23   Answer C

The language used is contemplative, serious and somber. Death is personified as the brother of Sleep to bring about a hopefulness of similarity. The description is vivid but rather intellectual and distant. Meredith thinks that Death should behave as a gentleman – consider the repetition of the phrase 'the decency of Death' which he regrets will elude him.

24 Answer D

The candidate should again see the irony of the situation – a man facing his own death sitting in the 'thin spring' (just about the beginning of life) sunshine, where there is so much life e.g. the courting couple (just about to begin their relationships). Consider the alliterations, the present participles like 'watching' and 'trotting'

25 Answer D

This can be seen from the words: 'It was difficult for Crooks to conceal his pleasure with anger.'

A man who lives in a room all by himself as a form of segregation in the ranch would feel loneliness but this is not the reason for his present hostility.

He does not feel embarrassed as it is the other two who have invaded his 'home', most likely because they felt lonely, too. He certainly is in no state of fear of these 'damaged' men.

26 Answer C

The fact that Crooks says that everyman has land in his head would suggest that it is a deep desire for humans to better their life chances and be better humans.
Answer A is too superficial even if true. Answer B may be true but does not capture the spirit of the passage. Answer D is suggested and comes close but even drifters have a longing for roof over one's head. Nonetheless, the crux of the answer is what is implied in the passage by the desire that each of these powerless men has articulated.

27 Answer D

The word 'selfhood' embraces all three of the other answers as selfhood means the state of being an individual. Each person desires to have a 'place they can call their own' which gives them a sense of independence and worth. It also means that a man has a roof over his head. It also means that he can have a family if he wants to and no longer need be single man. To have aspiration is an affirmation of the human spirit.

28   Answer **B**

Although the passage reveals Crooks to be brutally cynical, he nevertheless has an inner and deep desire for connectedness and friendship. Further he feels that he will be accepted by Lennie (and George) and Candy as they all are powerless men, alienated and lonely.

29   Answer **C**

Steinbeck has subtly revealed to the reader the status of these men and by demonstrating their needs and inner simplicity for connectedness and the need to connect themselves to land, shown his compassion and understanding. His philosophical concern is the affirmation of the human heart by focusing on social issues of the poor, the marginalised, discriminated and the old.

30   Answer B

The passage is spaced in the time of the industrial revolution in England which had a tremendous impact on Britain bringing technological, socioeconomic and cultural change to the nation. William Booth is focusing on the serious social problems such a vast change brought in its wake. From the passage, the candidate will gather that William Booth believes it is the neglect of authorities that such a horrendous situation arose in England.

31   Answer A

Booth took the opportunity of the news item regarding Stanley's visit to 'Darkest Africa' and used the descriptions of dense forests as analogous to the darkness in the lives of the poor working class. This analogy would draw sympathy or arouse a sense of anger at the social injustice suffered by the workers and the poor with its numerous comparisons of likenesses.

32   Answer D

Booth believed it was an impossible task to care for the population because of 'the innumerable adverse conditions' which overwhelm the reformers. Still keeping to the forest analogy, Booth states: They are battling against 'ten thousand million trees'.

33 Answer B

Paragraph two consists of several rhetorical questions which gives a cue as to the author's desire for his audience to hear his compassion and frustration about the plight of the unfortunate. He wants his listeners to think about the subject, about the world as a 'slum', as 'a purgatory'. His subject also touches on those who are social reformers and their desperate task. Thus a tone of frustration and compassion is aroused in the passage.

34 Answer B

Booth is concerned about the physical as well as the mental impact of the factories on the workers – 'the vice and poverty and crime' and the adverse conditions. He endeavours to draw attention to these problems by charging the people responsible for the state of the nation. There is no mention of the specific people responsible for righting these problems – people with a voice such as the church and those who have reaped the wealth as a consequence of industrialization. So eliminate D. There is the extended analogy of the forest but this has a function – it is not merely a comparison. Nor is the passage only a description of the weak and exploited – it is more intentional than that. Eliminate C.

35 Answer D

The cue to this is the line 'I believe that here it is a question of cruelty used well or badly' and Machiavelli goes on to illustrate his notion of the methodology a prince must use. These are pragmatic in the sense that he is dealing with the question of how society is run.

36 Answer B

The cue to this answer is in the sentence: 'Above all, a prince should live with his subjects in such a way that no development, either favourable or unfavourable, make him vary of his conduct.'

37 Answer C

Violence is used but only once and for all (That means make it count, after summing up the initial necessity to do so). It is imperative to do D. Conferring benefits is to be done gradually ('in that way they will taste better')

38 Answer D

It seems like raw political power to use advocate cruelty, but Machiavelli qualifies this type of conduct. He is promoting strategies of statecraft but these would be worthless without a skillful, effective, rational and pragmatic leader, who in turn is the personification of the good of the state.

39 Answer B

The clue to this is in the first sentence : the obstacles to their preservation .... prove greater than each man's strength to preserve himself in that state.
Rousseau has not touched on law-making or rising population or group-formation yet. Thus A, C and D can be eliminated.

40 Answer B

The phrases 'a form of association', 'defend each member with the collective force of all' and 'obeys no one but himself' and 'remains free as before ' are the principles of a social order which Rousseau ultimately wishes to see built. To do this there must be a social contract.

Nowhere does Rousseau state that it is imperative such a contract means all individuals merely have to obey the legal structures. C and D are very weak and inadequate answers. Eliminate as there is insufficient foundation for these.

41 Answer D

Answer A is tenuous as a social contract expects solid principles. Eliminate.
Answer B is not true as nowhere in the extract does it indicate that Rousseau's concept is a police state. C is a superficial interpretation of the question. Delete.

42 Answer D

'The articles of these contract are so precisely determined' Rousseau states, so that there will be nothing that might endanger it. All members are voluntary members. If a member contravenes his obligation, he goes back to the state of nature, so to speak, has a sort of anarchical freedom but loses his social freedom. Thus, the social contract is carefully tabled and would not include any rules that would mar its workability.

43 Answer A

The individual, according to Rousseau, has membership in a society based on a basic agreement that all are willing to agree to: that is, to transfer all their rights to the whole community unconditionally. In this way, Rousseau argues, everyone is under the same conditions and no one is above another. It is not illegitimate to do this. Thus B can be eliminated. Nor is the individual estranged as there is an association of all and Rousseau asserts that 'the union is perfect.'(paragraph 7). The collective body, or the state exists for the protection of the people (paragraph 9) – not to usurp their rights. So eliminate D.

44 Answer D

Everyone wins in this social pact. A social contract mandates specific behaviour that must be agreed to. Any obligation, either implied or explicit, that can be accepted or rejected, is a contract. In the social contract, the people and the state have a thorough obligation towards each other, as do the citizens also have mutual obligations to one another.

45 Answer A

The general will is the incorporation of 'each person and his powers' into the body politic for the common good.

46 Answer B

Thoreau is aware that government cannot be completely abolished or the result will be anarchy. It is not practical nor indeed, possible to return to a 'state of nature'. The second line gives a clear indication of the answer.

47 Answer C

The principle of self-determination is advocated here, where right and wrong are not decided by the majority but by the individual conscience. Eliminate A as Thoreau is critical of majority rule. As for B, the rule of law can be in opposition to the individual's conscience and Thoreau argues that a citizen should not resign his conscience to the legislature. D has not been a clear point in the argument.

48 Answer **A**

This answer covers all the other three – A, B and C.

49 Answer **A**

Thoreau is talking about each individual – that in a case of injustice, he should have the courage to stand up and be counted. This is a strong value espoused by any movement in search of reform

50 Answer **D**

Thoreau's argument is respect for the right rather than respect for the law. D is not in his argument.

51 Answer **C**

The line which provides the answer to this question is 'they have been effective in quenching and stopping inquiry' (line 3). By 'quenching and stopping enquiry', Bacon is referring to the stifling of desire to improve upon established knowledge. Bacon is not concerned with 'education' as such, but rather knowledge in itself, making answer (D) incorrect.

52 Answer **B**

These answers are other ways of stating 'uncertainty and fluctuation of mind', 'hatred of the ancient sophists',' and 'a kind of fullness of learning'. Reason (I) would appear to be logical and yet Bacon never cites poor education, but rather refers to a 'fullness' of learning, this illustrates how important it is to engage with the context of the language Bacon uses.

53 Answer **B**

Line 17 points out how the Greeks' occupied a middle ground between the extremes he has described in the earlier part of the text. Bacon does not refer to extremism in other matters, discounting answers (A) and (C). In answering, it is important not to apply Bacon's theories to anything other than what he discusses.

54 Answer **D**

The lines which support these two answers are, 'made everything turn upon hard thinking and perpetual working and exercise of the mind' in which we are encouraged as readers to admire the methods of the ancient Greeks' and 'was to be settled not by arguing, but by trying' in which Bacon makes his key point – that perpetual trying is the key to knowledge. There are no reasons to believe there is anger or any insult implied in the text, the tone is consistently placid. While Bacon admires the methods of the Ancient Greeks, this is clearly not the main aim of the piece as his focus is firmly on the process of deciding whether or not anything can be known.

55 Answer **A**

By describing a situation which will never happen (a shrimp whistling) and likening it to abandonment of the teachings of Marx, Engels and Lenin, the speaker makes his point very clear. (B) comes a close second but 'stop the teaching' implies educational teaching which is not the right contextual meaning of the quotation.

56 Answer **C**

The key to this quotation is understanding the contrast between 'discourse' and 'oration'.

57 Answer **B**

This statement requires careful thought. It uses the house as a metaphor for science, rather than suggesting that they actually are similar. (A) is too specific and is reading more into the comment than is actually there.

58   Answer **B**

The aim of this statement is to say that science cannot explain everything, and Einstein does this by giving the example of first love. (C) misses the main point of what Einstein is saying, his reference to the theory of relativity is merely a passing mention.

59   Answer **C**

This answer requires careful consideration of the quotation. 'One swallow' is a metaphor for a small hint of some future event, and we are urged to note that this one swallow is not definitive proof of summer - therefore we should not assume a small hint of some future event is its arrival.

60   Answer **C**

The easiest way to deduce this answer is by looking at the language used. The first few words, 'the most valuable result of all education' indicates that (C) fits best. Self-motivation is implied by the phrase 'whether you like it or not'.

61   Answer **C**

Using science 'more doors can be opened than with bare hands'. (D) that science breeds arrogance, is only very slightly implied by the quotation.

62   Answer **B**

Candidates will have to make a difference between The USSR which was a conglomerate of states under Communist Russia and present day Russia.
A can be eliminated because there is no indication of this in the cartoon
B The cartoon shows. Bush and not Putin driving – so it implies that he would like Putin to base his administration on western (American) style democratic ideas. On the other hand, Putin is referring to 'soviet model' which surely cuts against the grain of Bush's democracy.
C Russia is no longer a communist country. D we do not have indications of 'slow to remodel'.

63 Answer **C**

A is not sufficiently accurate. The cartoon is on the medico-legal and ethical aspects of any future need of the couple as well as the public focus on such a step because it is medical technology in practice.
B These two statements together do not cover the attitude of the cartoon or its intention. The simple union of two people is now a wholesale intrusion by many in so many fields of expertise.
C covers all the areas that the cartoonist is targeting – the private has become the public, IVF is complex in more sense than one, and the couple, before they even need to contemplate such a step, must foresee the invasion of all fields of experts into the lives. The cartoonist has drawn all these people crowding around the couple. Such is the 'modern love story'. Two have become an unwanted crowd!
D can therefore be eliminated as an insufficient message.

64 Answer **D**

The cartoonist is satirising the policy as one that has inherent contradictions such as 'cranking up more road hogs' and then 'abandoning the automobile'. It does not seem to be well-thought out as car assembly lines will only function when oil is struck. Also, the last panel states 'Go to 1' that is, the policy, finding no appropriate solutions is back to square one. This phrase seems to remind one of a game of snakes and ladders ie a game of dice!

65 Answer **B**

The 'old food pyramid' refers to nutritional guidelines which was supposedly the optimal consumption of food classes such as carbohydrates for all humans. It was neither sadisaster nor was it totally unworkable. Delete. It only is outdated when a new idea comes into existence but option A is vague.

66 Answer **B**

The comment can be taken as a slant of the government who cannot leave individuals to choose. It is meant as a jibe at authoritarianism. At the same time, there seems to be too much shifting from one line of thinking to the next so that the individual is left confounded.

67 Answer C

The cartoonist draws the attention to the terrorism in Zimbabwe by showing Western forces very obviously bypassing the African country in favour of bombing Iraq and Afghanistan, highlighted by the caption. Answer (A) is incorrect because the cartoonist has drawn what he sees happening at the present time, the attention of the West is bypassing Zimbabwe already. Answer (B) is incorrect because the cartoonist clearly feels the eyes of the world should be more focused on Zimbabwe than they are. Answer (D) is incorrect because the cartoonist clearly feels that there is something wrong with the current state of affairs - he is pointing out injustice (there would be no point in drawing a political cartoon showing things as they should be), therefore he cannot be suggesting that Zimbabwe should be left alone.

68 Answer D

The cartoon makes it visibly clear that military attention is on Iraq and Afghanistan and not Zimbabwe. Answer (A) is incorrect as the cartoon does not go so far as to directly suggest that the wars in Iraq and Afghanistan are pointless, or shouldn't be fought, rather his focus is on comparing these conflicts with Zimbabwe which is being overlooked. Answer (B) does not go far enough, the cartoonist does not simply feel that Iraq and Afghanistan are attracting too much attention; a key part of his statement is that the attention should be on Zimbabwe. Answer (C) misses the point of the cartoon. Whether or not the cartoonist feels the conflicts in Iraq and Afghanistan deal with terrorism is irrelevant compared to his assertion that Zimbabwe should not be ignored.

69 Answer B

The carton uses this caption to refer to Iraq and Afghanistan, where we are aware of attempts to fight terrorism, and then draws our attention to the over-looked situation in Zimbabwe. Answer (A) is incorrect due to the fact that the 'War on Terror' is not being fought in Zimbabwe; we know this from the planes in the cartoon passing over it without any action, compared to the bombing of Iraq and Afghanistan. Answer (C) is unsubstantiated. While the caption does contain an over-used phrase, its purpose is to more than simply mock it. Answer (D) is incorrect because the cartoonist does not directly blame the Western forces for terrorism, but rather points out the fact that they are ignoring terrorism in Zimbabwe.

70   Answer B

The tone is political - dealing with war, terrorism and the issue of where Western forces should be as well as raising questions about the legitimacy of political systems in Zimbabwe. The tone is also uncompromising - it makes a very clear point, not allowing for ambivalence. It is assured and decisive. Answer (A) is incorrect because while the message of the cartoon may be innovative, it is intended to make a serious political statement and does not use humour to do this in the way that other cartoons may. Answer (C) is incorrect because while the cartoon is very serious (solemn), dealing with serious issues, it is far from conservative, standing out against accepted policy. Answer (D) is also incorrect because the tone of the cartoon is measured and purposeful, without anger. While the message is political, it is not necessarily revolutionary in nature.

71   Answer C

This question addresses the irony in the cartoon and sums up why the cartoonist has used each of the elements in the cartoon - Zimbabwe, Iraq and Afghanistan as well as the visual image and the caption. Answer (A) is incorrect because the cartoon, while pointing out the discrepancies of the 'war on terror', does not completely dismiss the idea; rather it seeks a more balanced perspective. Answer (B) is incorrect because the fact that the planes are bypassing Zimbabwe is indicative of the fact that at the moment, the war on terror is bypassing Zimbabwe - the cartoonist feels it should not be. Answer (D) is also incorrect because the cartoon does not necessarily seek for an end to the wars in Iraq and Afghanistan, merely an end to the bypassing of Zimbabwe.

72   Answer B

The child's ancestry is discussed as if to give him a sense of identity but rather than describing cultural or ethnic origins, the father is focused on management and labour. The humour arrives from replacing one with the other in an unexpected way. (A) is incorrect as the there is no indication that the child does not understand what is being discussed. (C) is incorrect because the father is not obviously dismissing the child's grandfather. (D) is incorrect because there is not necessarily humour inherent in the idea of a child asking about his background.

73   Answer C

Statement II is correct as it is clear from the expression of the father that he is proud of his background, statement IV is correct because the father has replaced terms of ethnicity with those of occupation, Statement VII is correct because he father is eagerly placing a lot of importance on sharing what he perceives to be the child's heritage with him. Statement I is incorrect because this small episode is not enough to allow us to define the father's parenting skills on way or another. statement III is incorrect because the father, while pacing great importance on occupation, cannot be assumed to feel that it defines his family's future. Statement V is incorrect because the father's speech is not necessarily intended to indoctrinate the child as this response suggests.

74   Answer B

The fact that some animal has been killed on the road due to a literal U-turn mirrors the risk of damage to the public by figurative U-turns. Answer (A) is incorrect because although the cartoon deals with the unpredictable actions of the Government, it doesn't necessarily imply that their actions are irrational, merely changeable. Answer (C) is incorrect because it is limiting. The cartoon is a joke about the Government, but that does not mean the same thing as stating the Government is a joke itself. Answer (D) is incorrect because while the cartoon does imply that the Government's actions are changeable and therefore difficult to follow, they are not necessarily underhand or shady.

75   Answer C

The cartoonist is making fun of the Government's 'u-turns', that is their habit of making a decision and then changing their mind, going back on their word in a figurative U-turn much like the car which has killed the hedgehogs' companion in the cartoon. Answer (A) is incorrect because the cartoon does not deal with how the Government treat the public, but rather how they make their decisions. Answer (B) is incorrect because we are not given much of an idea of how the public react to the Government. Answer (D) is also incorrect because it is not the solidarity of officials which is really called into question, but rather the steadfastness of the decisions they make.

76 Answer **A**

The hedgehog characters are most definitely bemused, or puzzled, by what is going on. They are not directly affected; they represent members of the public. Answer (B) is incorrect because the hedgehog characters have not made any kind of stand against the government, they are bystanders. Answer (C) is incorrect because we are not mean to assume the country is truly run badly and also because the cartoon does not imply that the hedgehogs have been treated badly, merely that the death of their companion was an accident, for the same reason, answer (D) is also incorrect.

77 Answer **D**

The hedgehogs in the cartoon represent the public and they appear to express confusion and worry, wonder and concern. Their reaction is not extreme, or out of proportion, discounting answer (A), they are far from amused, discounting answer (B), and they are not obviously angry, discounting answer (C).

78 Answer **B**

The humour of the cartoon is aimed at the Government's decision making process. Answer (A) is incorrect because it is the decision-making which is ridiculed, not the nature of the decisions themselves. Answer (C) is incorrect because the cartoon is not dealing with any one aspect of policy. Answer (D) is incorrect because the humour is directed at the Government, not those who react to it.

79 Answer **C**

The unlikelihood of such a speech in a typical office environment. (A) is incorrect as the cartoonist is not merely making the speaker appear stupid, he is using him to point out the real attitude of management. (B) is incorrect as while the expressions are bewildered, this is to make the cartoonist's point - how unlikely an attitude the speaker has. (D) is also incorrect because the cartoonist is using the speaker in a sarcastic way, not realistically.

80   Answer D

The speaker's words are to be taken sarcastically to mean that warmth and decency are not the uppermost concerns in business. (A) is incorrect because the aim of the drawing is not to frown upon such a business, but to suggest that it doesn't exist. (B) is incorrect because there is no suggestion how businesses should act, just a reflection of how they don't act. (C) is incorrect because the aim of the cartoon is very much the opposite - to point out the colder side of capitalism, not highlight any warmer side.

81   Answer D

The cartoon is not merely suggesting a mistake has been made (answer C) but highlighting the irony of the recent decision. Answer (A) is incorrect because any humour in the cartoon is derived from the irony of the minister's speech and not at the expense of the homosexual. Answer (B) is incorrect because although the cartoon deals with the issue of balanced family life, it is more focused on what the Government has recently decided regarding same-sex partners providing that balance.

82   Answer A

The cartoon's main point is that a same-sex couple is logically not as damaging to a child as a same-sex institution. By making this point, the cartoonist is stating that the homosexuality of the parents is irrelevant compared to other parenting issues. Answer (B) is incorrect because the cartoon is more against the Government minister than the homosexual. The cartoon does not imply that the Government should stay out of the issue, as in answer (C), Answer (D) is incorrect because there is no implication that the government believes that being adopted by a homosexual couple is equal to encouraging homosexuality.

83   Answer D

The cartoonist points out the flawed thinking of the Government ministers by comparing the alternative to same-sex couple adoption favourable to a same-sex institution. Answer (A) is incorrect because although the cartoon is critical of the ministers' decisions, it does not state anything which actually suggests they are old fashioned or out of touch, even if this is implied. Answer (B) is incorrect because the cartoon does not go as far as to suggest that the Government decision poses a danger to children, merely that the decision does not make sense and does not benefit children. Answer (C) is also incorrect because the cartoon is more in favour of the homosexual than the children's home.

84   Answer D

The cartoonist clearly feels that being locked away in a same-sex environment until a child is grown up is worse than being adopted by a same-sex couple. This discounts answers (A) and (B). Answer (C) is incorrect because the cartoonist does not suggest that Government ministers should not be the ones to make such decisions but rather that in this case they have made a decision which does not make sense.

85   Answer B

The cartoon is pointing out the irony of the Government Ministers' decision - highlighting how nonsensical it is. Answer (A) can be discounted because although there is humour, the cartoon is actually raising a serious issue; it is in no way flippant. Answer (C) is also incorrect because although the cartoon may take a negative stance about this issue, its humour prevents it from being completely pessimistic or world-weary. Answer (D) is incorrect because in order to be activist the cartoon would have to clearly suggest and promote another course of action as an alternative to that which it is criticising.

86   Answer C

The dog and boyfriend are in each other's roles (it would make more sense if the boyfriend was inside telling the woman to go play with the dog as she wanted one). (A) in incorrect because we are not given any idea of what the cartoonist feels the typical dog's personality is - he has swapped him with the boyfriend. (B) is incorrect because the tone the cartoonist endows the dog with is not dominant, rather tired. (D) is incorrect because it is clear the woman owns the dog and the man is an adition to their party.

87   Answer B

The 'couple' in the cartoon are the woman and the dog, they treat the boyfriend as a pet. (A) is incorrect because while the man here is surplus, it is because the 'couple' have bored of him. (C) is incorrect because we do not hear from the woman in the cartoon and so her feelings can only be guessed. (D) is incorrect because while the woman has grown tired of her new boyfriend, this is not the main concern of the cartoon, it is clear that there is more going on than simply her bowered with her partner.

88 Answer **D**

The examples given of restrictions on Australian beaches are exaggerated for humorous effect. They have been embellished in order to highlight how ridiculous real restrictions on beaches have become. Answer (A) is incorrect because the cartoon is referring only to beaches and not necessarily to life in general. While the concept of diminishing freedom is crucial to the cartoon's message, the aim of the cartoon is not to make a general statement but to highlight a specific issue. Answer (B) is incorrect because the cartoon is making fun of health and safety rather than promoting it. Answer (C) could be considered correct but the cartoon is doing more than suggesting that the beach guidelines are hampering enjoyment - it aims to point out the foolishness and irony of the signs (for example a sign which warns the reader not to trip over the signs).

89 Answer **A**

The 'nanny state' describes a state in which the people are cared for like children, without any credit for common sense. The vast arrays of signs the couple in the cartoon are faced with assume they have no common sense and are over-cautious to the extreme. Answer (B) is incorrect because although there is a degree of paranoia in the nature of the signs (expecting something will go wrong), the cartoon is pointing out the unlikelihood of these signs proving useful, i.e. the unlikelihood of natural disaster. Answer (C) is incorrect because the signs in the cartoon do not reflect the public's opinion, but rather the authorities. Answer (D) is incorrect because there is no mention of compensation claims even though the signs are clearly a misguided attempt at health management.

90 Answer **A**

The cartoonist is being extremely sardonic (disdainfully or cynically mocking) and very sharp. Answer (B) is incorrect because the cartoon has a purpose, rather than being silly or pointless. Answer (C) is incorrect because the cartoon has a sense of fun and humour, it isn't strained or tense. While the cartoon aims to make a valid social point, it is not so extreme as to be considered radical, discounting answer (D).

91 Answer **D**

The humorous signs and exaggerated messages point to how outlandish the cartoonist feels the recent censorship is. The other answers are all incorrect because the sense of oppression, the idea that it could be detrimental or irritating is undermined by the humour.

92 Answer **C**

The signs are exaggerations of the sort of signs which have been seen on beaches. This is clear from the nature of the messages they contain, they are heightened versions of often-seen warnings. Answer (A) is incorrect because the cartoon is in response to a genuinely increased number of signs on beaches. They have not been merely imagined as this would make the cartoon pointless, so answer (B) is incorrect. Answer (D) is incorrect because the cartoon is very specific to its context - the characters are clearly on a beach and we are told that the cartoon was drawn in response to increased restrictions on beaches.

93 Answer **C**

Statements I and V are correct; the main feeling in the cartoon is that of isolation, and the fact that the lack of conversation is being celebrated is proof that a quiet, insulated workforce is considered good. Statement II is incorrect because there is no evidence of the workers feeling demoralised, statement III is incorrect as there is no mention of office politics, I.e. a row or conflict having taken place to cause the silence. Statement IV is incorrect as the cartoonist draws our attention to the boring, blandness of the office as if to highlight how soulless it is, it is not portrayed in a positive light.

94 Answer **B**

The sign on the wall should read something like 'number of days without a complain' or 'number of sales'; by making it about lack of conversation the cartoonist uses surprise to create humour. (A) is incorrect because the concept of such a soulless workplace is conjured up but does not evoke humour. (C) is incorrect because the prolonged silence is there to serve the prupose of the cartoon - to make a comment on the modern office. (D) is incorrect because the cartoon does not show the silence making life more difficult, there is no real argument for why it wouldn't work.

95 Answer C

Casting Nelson in the biblical role of Moses, parting the red sea, shows that the cartoonist thinks Nelson is over-confident. Answer (A) is incorrect because knowledge of the biblical story reminds the reader that the red sea was only held back for a short time and therefore Nelson's ability to hold back the cost of fuel will be short-lived. Answers (B) and (D) are incorrect because as we can see, Nelson is holding back the cost of fuel, albeit for a short time.

96 Answer A

Again it is the casting of Nelson as Moses which makes the cartoonist's message clear - Nelson posing as Moses highlights his self-assurance, clearly an over-confidence which cannot be substantiated. Answer (B) is incorrect because Nelson's power is shown to be short-lived - the tide can only be held back for a short time. Answer (C) is incorrect because the cartoon is not suggesting Nelson is blasphemous - casting him as Moses was the cartoonist's choice, not that of Nelson himself. Answer (D) is incorrect because Nelson is shown to be effective in the short term at holding back fuel costs.

97 Answer C

The tide will not be held back forever - therefore the riding fuel costs are inevitable. Answer (A) is incorrect because it is made clear that the rising costs are inevitable, unavoidable. Answer (B) is incorrect because although it is a reasonable assumption that the public would be frustrated by rising costs, this issue is not addresses by the cartoon. Answer (D) is incorrect because the biblical aspect is merely a metaphor; the morality of the issue is not addresses by the cartoon.

98 Answer D

The promise of Nelson to stem rising costs is shown to be an act of bravado which cannot last - therefore the warning against false promises closely matches the aim of the cartoon. Answer (B) is incorrect because having Nelson dressed and posing as Moses is sarcastic - we are being warned that he is over-confident, over-estimates his own power and therefore ewe cannot trust him. Answer (C) is incorrect because we are shown Nelson's ability to be working, for the moment anyway. The idea is that in time the prices will definitely rise, but for now he is holding them back.

99 Answer B

The metaphorical tide of rising fuel costs will crash down around the motorist at some point - therefore trusting Nelson could be a danger to the motorist as he will therefore be unprepared for the sudden rising costs. Answer (A) is incorrect because while financial issues are raised by rising fuel costs, the cartoon means to draw attention to Nelson's part in it all rather than the issue of costs itself. Answer (C) is incorrect because the tide in the cartoon is a metaphor for rising costs, not a literal tide. Answer (D) is incorrect also, this is because Nelson's power is not shown to be a risk to the Government or capable of causing major change.

100 Answer D

Statement I is correct because the cartoon is quite profound - it is characterising a modern problem - isolation. Statement II is also correct because as above, the male is thoroughly isolated and alone in his modern apartment. Statement V describes the irony of feeling lonely and rejecting company - the man turns away his caller because he has unnecessary things to do. Statement III is incorrect because the cartoon is not obviously humorous, but rather more disturbing- it is a social comment. Statement IV is incorrect because there is more of a sense of calm and depression than of chaos - the mans world is neatly ordered. Statement VI is incorrect because the cartoonist does not show the reader the consequences of refusing this offer of contact.

101 Answer A

The sense of dystopia comes from the misery of the character and the isolation which pervades the cartoon; it is recognisable and disturbing in it's evoking of real life. (B) is incorrect because there is a reason behind the depression evident in the cartoon - to define the modern man's isolation. (C) is incorrect because the piece is not intended to be comic, however keenly observed. (D) is incorrect because the cartoon may disturb but this is not equal to being actually repulsive.

102 Answer A

The third line in the first stanza says 'feeding a wife', 'satisfying a man', so the answer would include both the parents in the household.

103 Answer **C**

Parents adjust to any exigency ('involuntary plans') and in times of their kids' boredom ('dry hours') have to think of entertaining them in some way or other.

104 Answer **A**

A personification gives human characteristics to an abstract idea. Here dream 'flutters' and 'fight' (note the alliteration one a soft action and one an aggressive action). And dream can be talented and artistic – 'sing an aria'

105 Answer **A**

The speaker conveys feelings of despair because even if they had the space to dream in their lives-it would not come into fruition.

106 Answer **B**

The title tells the reader that the residence is puny. Rent is a factor that weighs on the minds of the personae and they are quick to ash for the bath while there still is warmth in the water.

107 Answer **A**

The past is gone and one cannot cling to impossible dreams.
Though all good things come to an end (D), this is too general in the context of the poem. Choose the more concrete and specific answer. Eliminate B and C as there is no indication of a broken relationship or an imminent death.

108 Answer **D**

There is no indication that the persona's youth is futile or that he is grateful that his life is ending. The poet is referring to the freedom of youth and all its possibilities. Consider the phrase 'free lances'.

109 Answer **A**

The sky signifies a vastness and a freedom that cannot be had when one's feet are on the ground. It symbolizes an escape from all restrictions and limitations. The church signifies religious and moral conventions- so both together symbolize an escape from the restrictions of life.
There was no hint of youth's ambitions. Eliminate C.
The sky's the limit is too colloquial. Delete B.
In this question, the candidate will need to go to a conceptual level.

110 Answer **C**

The word 'compels' is a very strong word, signifying that the earth is calling the persona. We remember the saying 'Dust thou art to dust returneth'. There is a certainty that cannot be denied.

111 Answer **D**

The persona is grateful for the thunder, rain and sunshine which symbolises all the good and difficult times in his life and for the opportunity he had to share his life with someone – maybe someone he loved. He thinks of these times with nostalgia – the tone in the closing stanza. A deep sense of fatalism is implied as well – in the line 'We are dying, Egypt, dying' and 'Not expecting pardon/hardened in heart anew.' The candidate needs to recognise all these elements which go to make this poem one of wistfulness, gratitude and acceptance of one's life forces.

112 Answer **B**

At first glance, it seems that A, C or D may well be an answer as the comparison of the squirrel to small coffee pot is indeed a cute and charming simile. But you need to look at the poem as a whole to realise the irony that cute seemingly harmless creature is utterly destructive.

113 Answer **A**

If you have answered the first question correctly, this question is not a problem. The grey squirrel has a hidden agenda as the words 'kills' and 'eats' will reflect.

114   Answer C

B seems to be a close answer but C is the answer, as the poet is targeting the concept of 'love thine enemies'. A can be eliminated as the poem does not touch on 'trigger-happy hunters' and no doubt he is performing a cull on squirrels, the poet does not touch on this either.

115   Answer B

A and D are ideas in the poem but the question asks the candidate about a 'twist' – that is the irony that the first part of the poem turns on. B can be eliminated as this is not part of the analysis of the poem.

116   Answer D

If you answered question 69 correctly then it should follow that you choose D as this is the second twist or irony found in this poem.

117   Answer A

118   Answer B

The cue is at the end of the poem where the speaker says 'old woman, /or nearly so, myself'

119   Answer A

The children did not comprehend the import of the lesson but the attitude was indifference.

120   Answer D

It was merely hypothetical so the children showed little enthusiasm

121 Answer C

The issue of what moral responsibility is

122 Answer C

There is a contrast brought about by time, the situation and whether a person is personally affected by the particular circumstances. At the present moment, time and a measure of wisdom have changed the attitude of the speaker C is the answer that covers these points.

123 Answer D

Time catches up with all things. The speaker has connected art, life and nature together in the inexorable march of time and now there is no question of being saved.

124 Answer A

The poet talks about herself spinning and Eve spinning because she wants the reader to make a connection between the first woman, Eve, and modern women. By doing this, she means to include all women in the poem. The poem does not just refer to one woman but the plight of women all through history. (B) is true to a degree, the poet is pointing out that women have to work hard, but speaking of Eve makes it clear she wants to say more than this.

125 Answer C

The lines 'For children gathered about our knees:
The thread was a chain that stole our ease' tells the reader that when the women have had children, they have felt bound by them. The word 'chain' suggests that the women feel tied or restricted by the responsibility of having children. It is important to look at a line from a poem in context - that is to read it and the lines which come before and after so you can gain a good appreciation of what the poet is trying to say.

126   Answer **D**

This part of the poem describes ways which the men have disappointed the women. We can tell this by the way in which the lines are written - the men have not lied or made mistakes, they are indeed 'strong', 'fond' and 'true' - but not in the ways which the women expected or not all the time. To answer this question it is very important to read carefully to appreciate poem's meaning.

127   Answer **D**

While (A) and (B) could be considered true, by describing the truth as a door which could be open and shut, the writer means more than just pointing out the man's dishonesty, he means the man's truth was 'open and shut', inconstant.

128   Answer **B**

The man returns from his wandering to find the woman there in order to comfort him despite his failings. There is no evidence that the woman feels comforted by the man and the poet does not suggest anything other than the woman being a comfort to the man. It is important in this question to look carefully at the language used by the poet in order to get the correct meaning of the words without making assumptions.

129   Answer **C**

The poem centres on the difficulties faced by married women. The key to answering this question is recognising that the poem comes from the point of view of a woman and therefore the reader does not get an idea of the man's feelings. For this reason (A), (B) and (D) do not truly describe the poem.

130   Answer **B**

By reading the description of the 'vast and trunkless legs of stone' it is made clear that the poet is describing a wrecked statue or sculpture. The shattered visage is therefore the stone face of the statue which we later learn from the description on the pedestal is Ozymandias. This question calls for a complete reading of the poem. It is important to read the poem a number of times before attempting to analyse it.

131 Answer D

The poet refers to the sculptor who carved the figure of Ozymandias. We know this from how he describes that the 'sculptor well those passions read / Which yet survive, stamped on these lifeless things / The hand that mocked them and the heart that fed'. It is necessary to read carefully and put the line into context - reading not just the line from the question but the lines before and after it.

132 Answer C

The poet focuses on how the statue of Ozymandias is ruined, despite the message on his pedestal. He tries to communicate a sense of what Ozymandias would have been like in life by looking at the expression captured by the sculpture. By describing how it has been destroyed he is telling the reader that Ozymandias was once great, but is no longer. This is the most important way that the poet wants the reader to think of Ozymandias - he puts a big effort into doing so.

133 Answer D

The poem clearly is making a very strong statement. We can work this out by looking at the points which the poet emphasises most; firstly the fact that Ozymandias was once a great leader, and secondly that now his empire has crumbled and there is only a worn away statue to his memory. This makes it clear that the poet wants to make a point about how man's power on earth (like Ozymandias' power) cannot last forever. While all of the other answers could be considered correct, they do not fully explain what the poet is trying to say.

134 Answer C

Ozymandias has claimed to be King of Kings and above the 'mighty', it is ironic that this message only survives in a desolate place written on a crumbling statue. It is common for a poet to end a poem by summarising his main theme. (A) is not quite correct because the poet does not want us to pity Ozymandias, we know this because of the way he describes him. Therefore we are not meant to pity him. (B) and (D) are not quite correct because although the poet does describe the desolation of the desert and the lonliness, it is not his intention to make this the focus of the end of the poem, he is describing the desolation of the desert in order that he may communicate a sense of irony to the reader.

135 Answer **B**

The poet dedicates the middle part of the poem to describing how well the sculptor captures the expression of Ozymandias, and remarks on this still being visible, 'frown / And wrinkled lip and sneer of cold command / Tell that its sculptor well those passions read'. (A) cannot be correct because we are not able to deduce if his work stood the test of time well as we do not know from the poem how long the statue stood for.

136 Answer **A**

Statement I, the poet tells us 'the old-time joys and faces-they were gone for many a day' - it is obvious from this line that the women had to leave loved ones behind. Statement V, the line 'The red sun robs their beauty' very clearly tells us that the women's looks suffer from their harsh lifestyles. Statement VII, it is clear that the women are far from female company, 'And there are hours men cannot soothe, and words men cannot say - / The nearest woman's face may be a hundred miles away.' This line makes it clear that they suffered due to this lack of female company.

137 Answer **C**

In the very first stanza of the poem the reason so many women left for the West is made very clear, in the line 'For love they faced the wilderness'.

138 Answer **B**

This line refers to the strength of the women as described in the poem. The intention of the last verse of the poem is to make it clear to the reader that the heart, or strength of the whole nation is a result of the hearts, and strength of the Women of the West. Answer (A) can also be considered true but in this particular line the poet uses the word 'heart' which points the reader to not just the physical body but the spirit and bravery of the women and the nation.

139 Answer **C**

This is the only phrase in which both words adequately describe the women based on what the poem actually tells us. Each of the other phrases has one or more words which do not describe the women well. For example (D), while the women may be considered lonely, they are not directly mistreated by anyone.

140 Answer **A**

The poet is paying tribute to the Women of the West by describing what they endured and admiring their achievements. This is made most obvious in the last verse when the poet links the strength of the women with that of the whole nation. The language of the poem makes the poets admiration clear, 'On the frontiers of the Nation, live the Women of the West'. (C) could also be considered correct but it is important to recognise that the poet is focusing on the feelings and experiences of the women. By doing this it is clear that the poet wants to do more than simply educate the reader. His language aims to make the reader see how strong the women were in order that we admire them.

141 Answer **C**

The line 'Four Seasons fill the measure of the year; / There are four seasons in the mind of man' makes the main theme of the poem easy to deduce. By dividing the life of a man into four seasons and describing how his mind is occupied in each one, the poet investigates the way a person's mind changes as time goes on and he becomes older. The poet does address the passage of time (B) and the fragility of life (D) but his focus is on how the changes of time infuence the mind.

142 Answer **B**

The line 'when fancy clear / Takes in all beauty with an easy span' suggests that the man in the 'spring' of his mind is imaginative (fanciful) and relaxed ('with an easy span'). (C) is incorrect because the term 'lusty' used here means eager. (A) and (D) can be considered fitting but they do not describe the mind of man in the way that the poet intends by his choice of words.

143 Answer B

To 'ruminate' is to muse over, or think fondly of and so it is clear that the poet means that in the summer of the mind the man thinks over his 'honied' (or sweet) 'Spring' (or youth). While (C) could be considered correct, the poet tells us exactly what the man is dreaming about and so it is not as complete an answer as (B).

144 Answer A

The line 'contented so to look / On mists in idleness--to let fair things / Pass by unheeded' tells us that the man in the 'Autumn' of his mind is happy ('contented') to watch the world go by 'unheeded'. We are not told of any sadness or laziness in the man, the term 'idleness' merely means the man is inactive, not lazy. The fact that he is 'contented' goes against the idea that he is tired out or sad.

145 Answer D

The final two lines of the poem, 'He has his Winter too of pale misfeature, / Or else he would forego his mortal nature' tell us that in the Winter of the man's mind there is nothing much to note - 'pale misfeature' and yet this final season in his life is necessary, because all men must die - this is their 'mortal nature'. It is important to look at the actual words chosen by the writer.

146 Answer B

Careful reading shows that the poet is describing the way 'fair' or beautiful thoughts run through the mind of the young man in a very natural, uncontrived way. The poet describes this by comparing the flow of thoughts to the flow of a stream near the beginning of its course. (A) and (C) cannot be true as the idea of letting things pass by is not the same as refusing opportunities or ignoring them.

147 Answer C

Answer A is too general because it does not take into account the writer's discussion of the reasons for this state of affairs. B is a close answer but it emphasises 'modernist culture' without a mention of the interface with the economy. D misses paying attention to the role of cuture (that is, artists and writers etc.) in society. Answer C covers Bell's discussion that in modern society, moral and character-forming strategies are neither given by capitalists as before, nor by cultural leaders and institutions as 'modernism has been trivialised'. Further, he remarks that 'the legitimation of social behaviour passed from religion to modernist culture'.

148   Answer   C

In the pursuit of wealth and pleasure, people have lost their spiritual basis. Matrial wellbeing is insufficient as a sustaining force in life.

149   Answer   C

Everything is produced by the economy to sustain 'lifestyle' which then becomes the differential between individuals. The market is the criterion of lifestyle. Experience is a means of pleasure and its boundaries become pushed to the limits – 'nothing is sacred'. A phrase like this gives the cue to the answer.

150   Answer   D

The paragraph explains itself.

151   Answer   A

All the examples given reiterates the author's implication for the counterproductive role of the media.

152   Answer   C

The continuous search for the limits of pleasure and lifestyle entails the pursuit of the new, the 'quirky and the aberrant'. It is as if modernist humans need to be continually on a high.

153   Answer   B

It is that in establishing new 'fads and fashions', these have then become the norm.

154 Answer A

A thorough reading of the extract suggests that the narrator is jealous of the woman she views through the window, Veronica, for physical reasons, 'her trademark red lipstick confusing, or perhaps accentuating, all the orchid delicacy she had going for her' and because of her career as a writer, 'Always canny, she discovered true crime sold better than fiction'. It is clear that she is paranoid from the way she feels it is necessary 'to seem natural and bright' and when she says 'I walked around my house as if visible from every angle; suddenly the walls were made of eyes'. The fact that she considers a fight between herself and Veronica is another strong clue that she feels both jealous and paranoid.

155 Answer D

It is clear that the narrator is a teacher , 'Turning back to the class, it was difficult to muster composure' and that Veronica is a writer, 'she discovered true crime sold better than fiction'. This question is straight-forward but highlights how important it is to read thoroughly and without jumping to conclusions.

156 Answer C

Veronica is described as having 'delicacy', and being 'thin and graceful', all of which can also be defined by the term 'dainty'. It is clear that she has been successful from the fact that the narrator has read her book. She is also described as strategic, which has the same meaning as tactical. It is important to look at what the words actually tell us. (D) is a close second choice but we are never actually told that Veronica is beautiful although it is implied, and the fact that the narrator feels threatened by her does not necessarily mean she is actually threatening.

157 Answer C

The key to answering this question lies in the next line, line 8, 'Except for Veronica' - it is clear the writer is trying to make the reader aware of how Veronica is different to the other mothers. While these lines do show the narrator's attention to detail this is not the main purpose of them.

158   Answer **B**

The story the passage relates is a clichéd story, typical of the sort Veronica used to read. We know this from reading line 26 when we are told that Veronica used to read parlour detective stories. The following lines must then be the narrators idea of what parlour stories are like; her tone is quite sarcastic.

159   Answer **B**

Veronica discovered that 'discovered true crime sold better than fiction' which tells the reader that it is real life crime which Veronica writes. The title of the novel which the extract comes from is also a clue to this - it is often extremely enlightening to read the title of a piece and keep it in mind when analysing it.

160   Answer **B**

In order to back up his claims that there is a large demand for historical information, the writer gives examples which he himself had a part in, thereby making his point clearer. There is no need otherwise for him to establish his credentials, therefore answer (A) is incorrect.

161   Answer **C**

The idea that political history will become more important as time goes by is suggested by the beginning of the piece when the writer excuses current ignorance by the youth of the nation, 'it might be the virtue of a still young country'. The writer suggests that the history of war, the military and sport are often uppermost in peoples' minds, but this does not equate to him placing them under political history in terms of importance, thus discounting answer (A). When the writer discusses other decades and the academic writing called for, it is with reference to contemporary history, not political history.

162   Answer **C**

In the first paragraph, the writer suggests 'we take too little note of political history, seeing war, military history and sport as closest to our identity'. The fact that he is keen to point out how political history is not generally considered a part of identity, and then the fact that he goes on to underline the importance of political history, we can deduce that the writer suggests a readdressing of identity in order to include what he feels is missing. Answer (B) is untrue – the writer feels there is a higher demand for history than is generally thought.

163 Answer **B**

A number of times Kelly sets himself up as an authority above another, 'I think there is a bigger market for Australian history than most publishing houses would believe', 'Federation, I think, has had a bad press for too long'. Answer a, while true, does not go far enough to describe Kelly's attitude and his main aim is not to share the experience he describes. While Kelly clearly wants to share his opinions, he does not give any reason why this is so, neither as a result of his experience (A) nor obligation (D).

164 Answer **D**

Kelly's main aim is to highlight the crucial importance of political history. He constantly refers back to the importance of history and the fact that history, specifically political history and especially the concept of Federation, deserve a resurgence in popularity. He feel that as time passes it is more necessary to value political heritage and so answer (C) is incorrect. He merely implies that people are becoming ignorant of their own heritage, admitting that other elements of identity are valued, making answer (B) incorrect.

165 Answer **A**

Key to answering this question is the recognition that Kelly aims to encourage the Australian to re-evaluate their appreciation of Australian history. It is therefore unlikely that he would insult his reader in the very first sentence, discounting answers (B) and (D). The sentence forms the introduction to the passage and is therefore intended to be witty rather than light-hearted. Although the line is something of a generalisation, it forms part of the writers argument and is meant to be taken seriously, not therefore a throwaway comment (C).

166 Answer **D**

The "deluded Irish"(line 5) convicts of 1791, who were ignorant enough to expect to find China by fleeing Australia overland through the bush, would have had little concept of China beyond such evocations.

167   Answer B

Line 14 shows Collins's "disapproval," which has a paternalistic quality, while he refers to the convicts as a group as "naturally vicious," a bigoted statement. Disapproval is not a quality that connotes fearfulness, though it could be argued that Collins suspected the worst of the "vicious" group.

168   Answer A

There are touches of dark humour, here (as in lines 12 and 13, "...three of them were so sure they had reached China...") and maybe a note of incredulity at the "magical" compass; but the author's language throughout the passage is for the most part free of direct judgment. He refrains from stating directly, for example, that Collins is a racist; instead he says "with his usual disapproval of the croppies" (line 14). And there is irony in many parts of this passage, for example, the naïve language the author employs in his description of the convicts' fantasy of the Orient: "... queer-looking blue bridges and willows just like the ones on plates..." (lines 2 and 3).

169   Answer C

Though any of the answers might be correct, it is likely that only liberty and life-threatening conditions (lines 3-5) would drive so many (line 20) to take the terrible risks Hughes illuminates throughout the passage.

170   Answer A

All the efforts of the escapees to reach China do, in fact, turn out to be futile. A compass without a needle is a guideless guide, and seems sure to result in a doomed journey. Leaving the reader with this last, powerful image, after the litany of examples of the convicts' failures provided by Hughes in lines 5-12 is a way of punctuating the hopelessness of their quest.

171 Answer **D**

Pyne believes it is "too much" to claim that fire was" the first phenomenon on which the human mind reflected," (lines 6-8), but agrees with Bachelard that it helped develop the human mind (lines 9-11). Throughout the passage, the author refers to the significance of fire in building the Aboriginal mythology, but he does not state it so emphatically as to claim it as the entire foundation for that mythology. He states, rather more cautiously, that it "was at least partially conceived and animated by fire (lines 1-2).

172 Answer **C**

All of these answers might be correct in other contexts, but the context in which we become acquainted with Bachelard in this particular passage involves a discussion of the mind and human intellect (lines 6-10).

173 Answer **C**

Fire, Pyne argues, at least in part, was a cause of the new patterns. As with dreams, the new patterns "relied on emotional or symbolic associations, without analogues in actual life" (also lines 16-17). Landscape is not referenced in this passage.

174 Answer **B**

Though one could infer that (A) and (D) could also be correct, the question asks the reader to look at the last paragraph for specific evidence. Lines 19-20 state that the new patterns not only created a new cognitive universe that helped form Aboriginal identity, but "a moral universe that informed him how he should behave."

175 Answer **A**

Though any of these answers might be true in and of itself, the question asks for a restatement of lines 20-21. Examining those lines closely for the same statement using different words will rule out (B), (C) and (D).

176 Answer C

The author mentions the community's "surreal whimsicality"(line 2) and "whimsy"(line 4), and the whole idea of a regatta or boating celebration in a dry river bed is absurd. Though the community may have a good business sense, driving them to hold the absurd event, it is after line 5 that the event is mentioned as a tourist attraction and a source of income for the town.

177 Answer D

"People in from the settlements on a temporary binge" are distinguished from "Aboriginal alcoholics and their families" in line 24. Lines 26-29 give evidence for the desperation of the Aboriginal alcoholics, certainly, but the question asks for evidence that the settlers' relationship is less so.

178 Answer A

In lines 27-29, the Keneally's quote seems to suggest compassion for at least the Aboriginal kid, if not his parents. (B) could also be correct, as judgment of the parents may be present in the man's statement; but given that the object of his statement is the kid and not the parents, (A) is the best answer here.

179 Answer C

(B) is very close to (C), but it seems that the main contrast here is between the Aboriginal and the white settler. The description of an irreverent and silly celebration contrasts mightily with the "hellish" existence of the Aboriginals. People in the relatively privileged position of taking out insurance against rain in a parched land and worrying about potential commercial disaster (lines 5-9) may face challenges of their own, but the plight of the Aboriginals as represented in Keneally's last paragraph does not allow much room for such celebrations (lines 20-21).

180 Answer C

Lines 24-26 state that the ordinance simply shifted the alcoholic populations to areas north or south of town, but does not state that the ordinance mitigated the inherent problems with alcoholism or the problems giving rise to alcoholism. One could argue that displacement could result in worsened conditions for the Aboriginal alcoholic families, thereby increasing their dependence on alcohol, but evidence for this is not given in the passage.

181 Answer B

The language used is not in keeping with Amy's narration and more in line with her accepted learning from her family, this is highly suggestive of the fact that she is quoting from a family member.

182 Answer D

Amy clearly revels in her description of how the victims 'burn visibly'. Her language shows he is attracted and fascinated by what is most likely her imagination running away with her. She has taken an abstract idea and made it very visual, there is nothing to suggest she is actually frightened.

183 Answer C

References to Sodom, 'he has practised abominations', his attempts to be frank and the fact that Amy as a ten-year old is not aware of the details of Charles 'sins' clearly point to his homosexuality and therefore the refusal of his family to accept him.

184 Answer C

The fact that the passage focuses heavily on the fact that Charles is only seen from a distance suggests the emotional separation as well as the physical distance between him and the family. The space is a metaphor for his exile.

185 Answer A

Amy's attitude to the men echoes her attitude to the victims of Sodom visibly burning - she is fascinated by them visually, noting details of their physical appearance and yet the details she focuses on are unattractive - grey toenails and hair. This is in keeping with the fact that she goes out on the farm with them and yet seems repulsed by their morning routine.

186 Answer A

The number of references to her family which Amy offers to confirm the religious ideas she has strongly suggests she has been indoctrinated. She uses phrases and refers to concepts she does not fully understand, hinting that she is merely repeating what she has heard in a way typical of her age.

187 Answer A

(A) political powers, is the correct answer. According to the selection, the Australian government instructed people to describe Aborigines as "aboriginals". The Australian government also wanted to limit the rights of Aborigines by choosing not to accept them as citizens, which was done by choosing not to capitalize the 'a' in aboriginal. Political powers were using language to limit the citizenship of Aborigines.

188 Answer C

(C) formal recognition of an indigenous people, is the correct answer. If the 'a' is capitalized it signifies the formal name of a group of people. Groups of people are recognized by the capitalization of their name. According to the selection, the Australian government was choosing to refer to a group of people as common nouns by not capitalizing the 'a', which limited their rights as citizens. By formally recognizing these people with the capitalization of the 'a' the government is indicating that they are citizens. (B) would not be the answer because capitalizing a name does not give the definition of a name. It only signifies its importance.

189 Answer C

(C) It diminishes their importance within a society, is the correct answer. When a noun is not capitalized it is seen as a common noun, such as book or cat. These common nouns do not have important significance. According to the selection, the Australian government was choosing to refer to a group of people as common nouns by not capitalizing the 'a'. Therefore, the word aborigine was no more important than a word like book or cat.

190 Answer D

(D) discrimination, is the correct answer. The Australian government was choosing to discriminate against the Aborigines by not recognizing them as citizens, which was done by referring to Aborigines as common nouns. (B) is not the correct answer because it was not a formal law to discriminate against the Aborigines.

191 Answer D

(D) formalize an identity, is the correct answer. Using the correct capitalization and adjectives will formally recognize Aborigines as a people. This will allow people to recognize Aborigines as citizen and address them in the formal manner they should be addressed.

192 Answer B

The suburbs may have been the great American fantasy, but looking at word choices in line 2, including the phrase "$250,000,000 planned community;" and the repetition of the words "sales," "brochure," and "developers," not to mention the litany of numbers throughout the passage, the idea of city as commodity is strongly suggested. Waldie opens the passage by saying, "…it wasn't a city at all;" and the aforementioned word choices also exclude (C) as a solid answer.

193 Answer D

(B) could be a correct answer here, but again, the repetition of numbers – and Waldie's choice of words like paved, concrete, light poles, etc. – give lines 3-5 a sterile, flat tone. A sense of alienation could certainly derive from the sterility of the picture.

194 Answer D

The purpose of advertising, after selling, is to extol the virtues and desirability of a product, and it is no different here in the lists of features of blocks, houses, and streets quoted throughout the passage. The claim that the community will be "the only garbage-free city in the world" is indeed absurd (line 11), but it would be absurd from our perspective or Waldie's, not the advertisers'.

195 Answer A

A synonym for "holy land" is "place of pilgrimage." Irony would be found in its opposite meaning. (B) and (D) have qualities antonymic to "holy land" and are therefore ironic.

196 Answer B

No judgment may be implied at all; but if it is, it is present in the structure and order of the list of denominations. Waldie may mention the fact that the list is not alphabetized to subtly hint at suburban religious bias of the times.

197 Answer C

A conversational tone can be detected in lines 1-3 and 6-10. Opening the passage with a question, and then pleading with the reader not to "think my reaction is the result of intolerance toward my neighbor" and discussing his own inadequacies with language are techniques that establish a relationship between Calvino and the reader. Though he is in a state of despair about human carelessness of language, he identifies himself with the rest of humanity rather than setting himself hatefully apart.

198 Answer B

It is the "random," "approximate," "generic" and "anonymous" that Calvino rails against in lines 4 and 15-18. (C) may also be correct, since Calvino protests the abstract, too; but it is specificity as well as dynamism that he seeks in Literature and in continual revision.

199 Answer C

When Calvino illuminates his own falterings with language (lines 6-10) it establishes an equality between himself and the rest of the world whose treatment of language he bemoans: "the worst discomfort of all comes from hearing myself speak." Thus it does not seem he is claiming superiority here. As a gifted writer capable of pointing out the vagaries of language, he is not claiming inferiority either. And, as the whole point of the passage is to defend the creative and cognitive use of language which is his passion and livelihood, Calvino does not seem to consider himself unusually particular or obsessive – though the reader uninterested in literature may.

200 Answer **A**

A best use of words makes (A) more correct than (D). It is our careless use of language Calvino bemoans, but our "distinctive faculty" is the "use of words" (line 13).

201 Answer **D**

Though Calvino exaggerates, and endears himself to us by stating that "the worst discomfort of all comes from hearing myself speak," (again, line 6) he elaborates on that initial statement by explaining that his reason for writing is to revise until he comes to a place of eliminating at least "dissatisfaction" with his expression of ideas (lines 7-10).

202 Answer **B**

The strangeness of unfamiliar landscapes and languages that Basso discusses at length and from the first lines are potentially "downright unsettling" (line 4), "remote and inaccessible, anonymous and indistinct" (lines 12-13), and "keenly disconcerting." The strength of these adjectives and the repetitive insistence of such ideas throughout the passage could lead the reader to believe Basso is describing personal experience as an alien in a new context. (C) may also be correct, but we cannot find direct evidence for this in the text, and Basso does not seem alone when it comes to being part of a group of ethnographers.

203 Answer **C**

Basso is willing to appear less than a perfect expert by admitting his alienation among the twin mysteries of unfamiliar landscape and language; indeed he introduces no real hypothesis here beyond the fact that this combination can be extremely disconcerting (ie., lines 1-4). It is not so just for him; he relates himself repeatedly to other ethnographers and strangers who may or may not be ethnographers (lines 8-9, 17). Therefore, though it may seem like (D) could also be a correct answer, it is not quite accurate, because the phenomenon Basso describes is personally experienced but also related to a universal experienceof being an alien and a stranger.

204 Answer C

All of the answers could be correct, here, but landscape and language are strongly linked in almost every line of the passage, and perhaps most forcefully in the first eight lines. Indeed, the first line of the passage opens by linking the two phenomena.

205 Answer A

According to these lines by Basso, the "stranger's efforts to invest" new landscapes and languages with "significance" is fruitless in trying to actually comprehend the new situation, and even accentuates his discomfort. One might extrapolate that, in order to connect with the new context, it would be necessary to enter and inhabit an entirely different mindset, one formed by the alien landscape and language. (C) might also be correct, but only independent of this particular question.

206 Answer D

"Determined" and "interested" are active states and qualities usually attributed to sentient beings, not landscapes or languages. In these lines, landscape and language take on an almost mocking quality. Lines 4-5 are close, but not quite anthropomorphized.

207 Answer C

The main point of the passage is that real-life detectives do not behave in the same way as fictional detectives. In describing fictional detectives as "individualistic", the author implies that real-life detectives are the opposite: in other words, they cooperate with others and prefer to work as part of a team. This rules out choice (A), since working without cooperation is individualistic behavior. It points strongly to (C), because accepting help from others is contrary to individualism. (B) is a poor fit because the author does not say that real-life cases are bizarre or difficult to solve. If anything, he implies that real-life cases differ from those found in detective mysteries. (D) may or may not be true, but is not addressed by the passage at all. The best choice remains (C).

208 Answer B

The emphasis of the passage is on the work done by police officers who are first to arrive at the scene. In fact, the second sentence states that "it is the actions taken by the patrol police who get to the scene first that determine the outcome." This indicates that (B) is the correct answer. (A) is not a good choice, because nothing is said about laboratory work here. (C) is irrelevant because lawyers are not responsible for solving crimes, and are not mentioned in the passage either. We can rule out (D) because the thrust of the passage is to minimize the work of detectives, emphasizing the work of patrol police who arrive first at the scene of the crime. (B) is by far the best choice.

209 Answer D

The passage is concerned with the privileges enjoyed by police detectives, and mentions the freedom to wear civilian clothes as one of these privileges. Wearing a uniform must therefore be something other than a privilege for a detective. This rules out choice (C). It also argues against (B), because even if the police uniform commands respect, the author is implying that it is more valuable for a detective to go without a uniform. The answer must be either (A) or (D). Let us first consider (A). Although the passage hints at the importance of working undercover, it does not mention the degree of danger faced by police detectives, and does not even imply that doing detective work in a uniform would be anything more than an inconvenience. Now look at (D). The passage does state that a uniform would identify the wearer as a police officer, implying that it is better to do without that kind of attention. The best answer is therefore (D).

210 Answer A

Choice (B) is incorrect because wearing casual clothes on the job is cited as a privilege of detective work. (D) is also wrong, since the passage does not say anything about the interaction between detectives and journalists. Instead, it mentions the similarly confidential nature of a journalist's contacts and a detective's informers. This leaves (A) and (C). At first glance, (C) seems to be appropriate because the passage comments on detectives keeping sensitive information secret from the boss. However, it also says that keeping secrets is a necessary freedom of detective work. It goes on to say that a specific way in which this freedom can be abused is if detectives pretend that they are working with informers when they are actually not working at all. This is the point made in (A), which is more specific than (C) and therefore makes a better answer.

211 Answer A

Choice (B) is a poor fit because Passage III is not arguing that real-life detectives are less intelligent than the fictional detectives described in Passage I. Passage III deals with morality rather than intelligence. In particular, it brings up the possibility of detectives avoiding their duties by abusing the confidentiality privilege that comes with their work. In saying of real-life detectives that "it is frequently hard to know if they are really on the job or not," Passage III draws a contrast with the "strong moral fibre" of the fictional detectives in Passage I. This points to (A) as the correct answer. (C) is wrong because the "reliable testimony" in Passage II refers to the credibility of witnesses and not to the truthfulness of a detective. (D) is also a poor choice, since Passage III does not describe detectives as unskilled. The best answer remains (A).

212 Answer D

The best answer is (D). all of the above because no single answer is sufficient. The author uses all three of these techniques. Winton details sea creatures and records the "clicks and rattles" within this seemingly silent world to evoke this atmosphere. He also describes his boat in the simile "like a party balloon" to emphasize Fox's distance from his boat on the surface. Finally, the author details how water pressure tightens Fox's skin, and currents sway his hair: the physical effects of the dive.

213 Answer C

Winton introduces the question of whether Fox will make it back to the surface alive with the phrase "Pressure tightens his skin". The other choices – (A), (B) and (D) – instead employ peaceful, almost lazy images: skin on water, the slowly shifting fish and the almost motionless boat.

214 Answer B

Fox seems to want to stay down below, but not because of any radical change in point of view. He shows no evidence of wishing to change his life (A) or to deliberately end his life (C). Nor does the author exhibit a background of risky habits (D) to account for Fox's dreamy descent. Rather, "the magnetic quality of the primal" -- an otherworldly pull rather than his own will -- seems to spur Fox's temporary, almost involuntary wish to remain in the underwater depths.

215 Answer **C**

(C) is the best answer because the oxymoron "poisoned and happy" is a contradiction in terms. The body is slowly being poisoned by the effects of underwater pressure while the mind blissfully ignores this slow dying. In answers (A) and (B), the language evoked by "delirium" and "thick" creates no underlying tension or contradiction. Furthermore, (D) ("his body still does the breathing for him") implies cooperation between body and mind, not tension.

216 Answer **A**

Fox is half in the world because he has nearly experienced death, but principally because he is still ecstatic at the thought of the beauty down below, underwater (A). It is as though half of him has not yet emerged into normal, daily life but is still dreaming of that other world. The passage omits any discussion of morality, as suggested by (C). Furthermore, the author offers little hint of an afterlife, so this makes (B) is an overstated, insufficient response. The emphasis on a physical source for the "tingling" produces an incomplete answer (D), not the best.

217 Answer **D**

One arrives at the solution by considering all 3 passages with special attention to lines 1-3, 13-15, 20-22 and 26-28. The author elaborately explains that real objects, places people and the mind are a part of the space that exist outside of the mind and that these same realities and images exist within the space contained in the mind. (C) would have been the second best answer; however, it is too simplistic and does not define what the author is actually trying to convey.

218 Answer **B**

One arrives at the solution by considering passage II lines 13-14 and passage III lines 24-26. The author explains in lines 13-14 that if an experience has not left a lasting impression that it will become vague and basically forgettable and then in lines 24-26 the author explains that, although we seem to forget certain experiences the images are still there but not as easily recalled as those images or experiences that have excited our minds or that have stood apart from the mundane allowing them to occupy the space in our mind where they are easily recalled. In these lines the author imparts the impression that if images or memories are of some import them we store or file them in a space of the mind that is more easily accessible. (A) would have been the second best answer; however, the author is much more focused on those images that are worthy enough to occupy space in the mind.

219   Answer A

One arrives at this solution by considering Passage I lines 4-7 and Passage II lines 15-21. The author explains that images stored within the mind that are remembered are perceived through a space that is not an actual space and in lines 15-21 the author elaborates on this theory in that the perceived space is simply the use of one's imagination which is not truly a space but an action of the mind that allows us to remember those images that are actual parts of the space in the mind. (B) would have been the second best answer; however, the author has at this point made it clear that, although, images are a part of a perceived space that in truth is not an actual space at all.

220   Answer B

One arrives at this solution by considering Passage I in its entirety. The author explains that through the experience of having visited the Soudan, he can easily recall the image which is valuable in itself as a map in returning to the Soudan. The ability to factually recall the way to a destination is very useful. (C) would have been the second best answer; however, knowing what a place looks like does not mean that one could find their way there. The author implies that he has already made a visit to the Soudan and in doing so he can imagine the place clearly which allows him to imagine the exact path that he took to get there the first time.

221   Answer C

One arrives at this solution by considering passage II lines 15-21 and passage III lines 24-38. The author explains in lines 15-21 that we use our imagination to recall the images within the space of the mind that allow us to re-experience particular moments or events and the author further elaborates in lines 24-38 that these images are what we have already experienced and, further, that each of these images and memories serve as a foundation of a greater framework or mass that will guide us in our observations and understanding of those experiences yet to come. (A) would have been the second best answer; however, the fact that all that we have known will directly affect all that we have yet to experience is not clearly made through this statement.

222 Answer C

'Gillard rejected the suggestion Labor has been rattled by a sustained attack from the opposition over the Government's petrol policy' (lines 1-3). The key to this question is in reading the question thoroughly in order to see that you can identify an accusation which has been denied. The suggestion that Labor has been 'rattled' amounts to an accusation, and by refusing it, Gillard is denying she is 'rattled' or disconcerted.

223 Answer D

'What has driven the Government in this period is... those important promises to help working families and individuals' Answer (C). could have been selected but the key is understanding that Gillard was discussing the current motivation of the government, not just reminding the public of old promises.

224 Answer A

'Ms Gillard defended FuelWatch, saying it was about monitoring fuel prices and enabling people to identify the cheapest petrol in their vicinity'. In lines 16-18 as in the rest of the article, Gillards main concerns are to defend the government's actions (defensive) and to explain them (elucidative). While she could be considered ready for a fight (pugnacious), she is optimistic rather than pessimistic. Her arguments are consistent and not changeable and she is loyal to her cause rather than perfidious.

225 Answer C

The topic is not completely ignored but rather 'sidestepped' so Gillard can discuss the voting public's attitude to climate change. The answer refers to line 26 where Gillard describes the attitude of the public to climate change.

226 Answer B

Often the title of a piece gives a good indication of what the main message or purpose of the article is, especially in newspaper articles. While the article does intend to educate the reader about current debates (A), more of the article is devoted to describing how Gillard, as a representative of the Government, has reacted to criticism than is devoted to simply explaining the debates.

Worked Solutions

227 Answer B

To be 'on the front foot' in this context is to be taking advantage of the situation. While the reader is made aware in line 7 of the fact that the Opposition has actually gained popularity, (B) encapsulates this fact and expands on it to include the wider implication that the Opposition is capitalising on the government's embarrassment in other ways.

228 Answer C

STEP 1=> What do you need to determine to solve the problem?
You need to determine what the lines that intersect at point B indicate by following them back to the correct scale.

STEP 2=> What relevant data provided in this problem are needed in order to answer the question?
The example given for point A is a guide to which scale is correct. Horizontal lines through point A are read off the Strontium Nitrate scale, Wood Meal percentage is read by following the line that goes downward and to the right, and Potassium Nitrate percentage is read by going upwards and to the right.

STEP 3=> Use the relevant data/ example to solve the question.
Reading horizontally from point B, the percentage for Strontium Nitrate is 70; reading down and to the right gives 20 percent for Wood Meal; reading upwards and to the right gives 10% for Potassium Nitrate.

229 Answer B

STEP 1=> What do you need to determine to solve the problem?
What a horizontal line indicates and what an open square means.

STEP 2=> What relevant data provided in this problem are needed in order to answer the question?
The key shows what different symbols mean. The scales and the example given show what a horizontal line indicates. Horizontal lines are percentages of Strontium Nitrate.

STEP 3=> Use the relevant data to solve the question.
A series of points on a horizontal line mean that the percentage of Strontium Nitrate is the same for all the points. An open square (from the key) means that a particular

mixture didn't burn. The line of open squares means that no mixture tested at 50% Strontium Nitrate burned. Further, the open squares above the horizontal line show that some mixtures with 60% Strontium Nitrate didn't burn.

Our conclusion is that mixtures with greater than 50% Strontium Nitrate probably won't burn. So (B) is the correct answer.
Note that (D) is wrong because although 50% Strontium Nitrate and 50% Potassium Nitrate is on the same line as the others, it wasn't tested (and isn't marked) so we cannot say for sure that it won't burn.

230   Answer A

STEP 1=> What do you need to determine to solve the problem?
You need to find a trend that allows us to infer what a mixture at point C will be like.

STEP 2=> What relevant data provided in this problem are needed in order to answer the question?
Mixtures closest to Point C have the most similar percentages of each ingredient. They should be the best guide to what a mixture at point C will do. Looking at those points and the key should tell us if there is a pattern.

STEP 3=> Use the relevant data to solve the question.
The points closest to C are marked either as not burning at all, or burning moderately with a strong color. So, the least likely properties of a mixture at C would be the opposite of these. Fast burning and weak color; (A) is correct.

231   Answer A

STEP 1=> What do you need to determine to solve the problem?
Information from the graph and key. The graph to determine any trends and the key to translate color and shapes into whatever matches the trend.

STEP 2=> What relevant data provided in this problem are needed in order to answer the question?
There is a line of blank squares that runs through point D. It indicates that mixtures with 20% Wood Meal (all those tested) didn't burn. Point D also has 20% Wood Meal.

STEP 3=> Use the relevant data to solve the question.
The other points next to point D show moderate burning and strong color. Point D should share characteristics with either the line of blank squares or moderate burning or strong color. Anything not in this set is unlikely. The only answer that has characteristics that match is (A).

232 Answer C

STEP 1=> What do you need to determine to solve the problem?
You need to see if any of the listed operations change the graph so that the relative amounts of the ingredients stay the same, but only total 90% instead of 100%.

STEP 2=> What relevant data provided in this problem are needed in order to answer the question?
Simply following the methods in each answer and seeing how the percentages of each chemical change. If they change to meet the new condition (the addition of 10% stabilizer), then that is a valid method. If none suffice, then the last answer would be the default.

STEP 3=> Use the relevant data to solve the question.
Moving upward on the graph increases the amount of Strontium Nitrate and moving downward on the graph decreases the amount of Strontium Nitrate. But each move changes the relative amount of the other two ingredients as well. Neither up nor down can be correct.

Multiplying each scale number by 0.9 changes (for example) point A into 72% Wood Meal, 9% Strontium Nitrate, and 9% Potassium Nitrate. These total 90%, which is what we want. The relative amounts of each hasn't changed, since we multiplied all the scales by the same factor. These are just the conditions we wanted, so (C) is correct.

233 Answer C

STEP 1 = > What do you need to determine to solve the problem?
How likely each product is to catch the maximum number of drug users.

STEP 2 = > What relevant data provided in this problem are necessary in order to answer the question?
Since false negatives allow drug users to remain undetected, the false negative rate for each test is the relevant parameter.

STEP 3 => Use the relevant data to solve the question.
From lowest false negative to highest, the ranking is: Gotcha, Catch-It, DrugsBegone.

234   Answer A

STEP 1 => What do you need to determine to solve the problem?
What percentages of false positives and false negatives will result from combining multiple tests.

STEP 2 => What relevant data provided in this problem are necessary in order to answer the question?
The percentages of false positives and false negatives for each of the listed products.

STEP 3 => Use the relevant data to solve the question.
For Gotcha, if the total number of tests is X, and of those Y are actually drug users, then the number of false positives (fp) will be 0.05(X-Y). The total number of false negatives (fn) will be 0.1(Y). This leaves 0.9Y as the total number of true positives detected.
The total expected number of positive tests (true and false) would be 0.05X + 0.85Y, and this is the number of people who will be retested with DrugsBegone. The number of fp on this subset is 0.02(0.05X + 0.85Y - 0.9Y) = 0.02(0.05X - 0.05Y) = 0.001 (X - Y). This is also the overall false positive rate, 0.001. This is a simple multiple of the the two fp rates given alone.

The overall fn rate will be those who were caught on the first test who were actually drug users (0.9Y) who now test negative with DrugsBegone 0.15(0.9Y) = 0.135Y. In addition, those that were not tested because they passed the Gotcha test in error, 0.1Y, mean that a total of 0.235Y are missed by this combination of tests. Answer (A), fp = 0.1% and fn = 23.5% is correct.

235   Answer D

STEP 1 => What do you need to determine to solve the problem?
The ratio of drug users who test positive who actually use drugs to the total number who test positive.

STEP 2 => What relevant data provided in this problem are necessary in order to answer the question?
The false positive and false negative rates for Gotcha and the background rate of drug use.

STEP 3 = > Use the relevant data to solve the question.
Gotcha has a 5% false positive rate and a 10% false negative rate.
In a population of 1000 (from this demographic) on average, 100 will be drug users and 900 will not.

Gotcha will show that of the 900, 5% are drug takers when they are actually not. This is the false positive rate and will show 45 people who are not really taking drugs as positive for drug use. Of the 100 who are drug users, 10%, or 10 people, will show 'clean' when they are actually using drugs. This is the false negative rate. So, overall, 45 + 90 will get a positive test for drugs and of those, only 90 will actually be drug users. 90/ (45 +90) = 0.666... which rounds up to 67%.

236 Answer B

STEP 1 = > What do you need to determine to solve the problem?
How many people out of a hundred who tested positive in question 3 will still show a false positive result when retested?

STEP 2 = > What relevant data provided in this problem are necessary in order to answer the question?
The chances of a positive test (in this population) actually being false (fp)- given in question 3 as 67%. And the fp rate for Catch-It.

STEP 3 = > Use the relevant data to solve the question.
Retesting the new population with Catch-It means using a new background rate of 67%. In this new population group (those who already tested positive with Gotcha) 67 out of a hundred will be actual users and 33 will not. Catch-It will show 6% false positive, so that .06 x 33 = 2 people out of a hundred that tested positive on Gotcha will show positive on Catch-It when they are in fact, clean.

237 Answer A

STEP 1 = > What do you need to determine to solve the problem?
How pre-screening affects who will get the second, authoritative test.

STEP 2 = > What relevant data provided in this problem are necessary in order to answer the question?
The false negative rate for each product determines who 'passes through' the initial filter.

STEP 3 => Use the relevant data to solve the question.
The lowest fn rate is for Gotcha, so this will pass the most drug users on for final testing. The fp rate isn't important in this question, as any fp will be caught by GCMS.

238   Answer A

STEP 1 => What do you need to determine to solve the problem?
How many employees (as a percentage) actually use drugs.

STEP 2 => What relevant data provided in this problem are necessary in order to answer the question?
The fp for DrugsBegone is 2%, the fn is 15%, the total number of employees tested is 1000 and the positive test results are 186.

STEP 3 => Use the relevant data to solve the question.
Let U mean actual drug users and C equal 'clean' (not drug users). The total number of expected positive test results is U − fn(U) + fp(C) = 0.85U + 0.02C for any combination of U and C.

U + C = 1000 and 0.02U + 0.02C = 20. This gives two equations in two variables:
186 = 0.85U + 0.02C
20 = 0.02U + 0.02C

Subtracting gives 166 = 0.83U and U = 200 as the estimate for actual users. This is 20% of the population under consideration.

239   Answer D

STEP 1 => What do you need to determine to solve the problem?
What genotype combinations will lead to only black puppies as offspring?

STEP 2 => What relevant data provided in this problem are necessary in order to answer the question?
We are told that any combination of genes with B will have a black coat. That and examination of figure 1 to see how genes combine.

STEP 3 => Use the relevant data to solve the question.
Since all puppies are black, all must have a genome of the type Bx (where x can be

either B or b). To guarantee that every puppy gets one dominant gene, at least one of the parents has to be BB. A parent that is BB can only contribute dominant genes to offspring. So, all the combinations that have a parent with BB would be possibilities. The other parent can be BB, or Bb, or even bb.

240   Answer A

STEP 1 = > What do you need to determine to solve the problem?
The genome for the unknown male dog.

STEP 2 = > What relevant data provided in this problem are necessary in order to answer the question?
The mix of color in the offspring and the color of the mother.

STEP 3 = > Use the relevant data to solve the question.
Since the mother is black, her genome is either BB or Bb. If her genome were BB, then all puppies she birthed would be black, but we are told that some are chocolate. Therefore, her genome must carry the recessive b. By the same reasoning, the father can not be BB and must be either Bb or bb. The punnit square for Bb and Bb is given in figure one and shows that when Bb and Bb are mated, only about one in four puppies should be chocolate (bb). This doesn't fit with the information about the mix of coat colors in the litter.

A punnit square with the other possible cross- Bb and bb however, gives a 50:50 split between black and chocolate puppies. This fits the given data much better.

241   Answer A

STEP 1 = > What do you need to determine to solve the problem?
The genomes possible for the grandparents of the litter described.

STEP 2 = > What relevant data provided in this problem are necessary in order to answer the question?
The fact that the grandparents only produced black puppies and the final mixture of colors for the second generation. Also, the fact that the parents of this litter were siblings.

STEP 3 = > Use the relevant data to solve the question.
Since the grandparents only produced black puppies, one dog would have to be BB. Since the second generation includes some chocolate dogs, and this trait could only

be passed along through the parents who got it from the grandparents, one of the grandparents has to have a b. This only leaves the combination of BB and Bb for the original pair of dogs.

Neither grandparent was yellow, and none of their direct offspring were yellow. Therefore, the only combination of E would have to be EE with Ex (where we don't know x yet). Because the second generation does have some yellow puppies in it, and the only way to get the recessive trait passed down would be from a grandparent, at least one allele in the grandparents has to be e. That means that the grandparents have to be BB, Bb and EE, Ee. Which dog has which can't be determined, so either combination of the two sets is possible.

242   Answer C

STEP 1 = > What do you need to determine to solve the problem?
The probability that a yellow Labrador and a chocolate Labrador mated together will yield only BxEx offspring.

STEP 2 = > What relevant data provided in this problem are necessary in order to answer the question?
We know that chocolate Labradors have bb and we are told that this chocolate Labrador has EE. We also know that yellow Labradors have ee.

STEP 3 = > Use the relevant data to solve the question.
The only missing information is the allele mix in the yellow Lab for B. If the probability we want is for a litter of all black pups, what we need to find is the probability that the yellow Labrador is BBee.

From figure one, the probability of BB is 1:4. The other possibilities are bB, Bb, bb.

243   Answer C

STEP 1 = > What do you need to determine to solve the problem?
The probability that 5 puppies will be black given the genomes of the parents.

STEP 2 = > What relevant data provided in this problem are necessary in order to answer the question?
The parents genomes are given and can be used to discover possible genomes for their offspring.

STEP 3 = > Use the relevant data to solve the question.
Since only one parent has the recessive allele for yellow, no puppies will be born with ee. Looking at figure one, we see that of the five possible genomes for the B allele, three are black and one is chocolate. That means that each puppy born has a 75% chance of being black.

Multiplying .75 for each puppy: $(0.75)^5 = 0.2373$ or about 24%.

244 Answer C

Question 1
STEP 1 = > What do you need to determine to solve the problem?
The linear distance between point F and the hilltop.

STEP 2 = > What relevant data provided in this problem are necessary in order to answer the question?
The map distance (2 cm), the scale on the map (1:25,000) and the elevations of each spot.

STEP 3 = > Use the relevant data to solve the question.
2 cm on a map of scale 1:25,000 would give a ground distance of 50,000 cm, or 500 m for the ground distance. The difference in elevation between the two points is 263 – 210 = 53 m.

The linear distance is the hypotenuse of a right triangle with these two distances as the other sides. So the correct answer is found from (linear distance)2 = 5002 + 532.

245 Answer A

STEP 1 = > What do you need to determine to solve the problem?
What do the contours indicate between point A and the spot elevation 537?

STEP 2 = > What relevant data provided in this problem are necessary in order to answer the question?
The contour line closest to A isn't labeled, but others, as well as the spot elevation allow interpolation.

STEP 3 = > Use the relevant data to solve the question.
The contour line closest to B is labeled 500, and the spot elevation is 537, so from the 500 contour line to the spot elevation is uphill. The spot elevation is a hilltop.

Travel from the labeled contour line toward A doesn't cross 4 intermediate lines, so A cannot be at 550, and the contour line closest to A must be 500 also. Travel from A to the hilltop would be generally uphill.

246   Answer B

STEP 1 = > What do you need to determine to solve the problem?
The elevations of point A and point B and find the difference.

STEP 2 = > What relevant data provided in this problem are necessary in order to answer the question?
Point B is shown next to a labeled contour line and between two labeled contour lines. This allows interpolation of B. Point A is next to a contour line but has no other slope information, so the range that point A can be is different.

STEP 3 = > Use the relevant data to solve the question.
Point B, by convention is at 495 m. Point A although next to another 500 m contour line, could be higher or lower-- the map doesn't tell us how the ground slopes in the area A is in. So, point A could be as much as 505 m and as little as 495 m. This means that the most point A and B could differ by would be 10 meters.

247   Answer B

STEP 1 = > What do you need to determine to solve the problem?
How high the tower must be so that the top is visible above the hilltop with elevation of 537 m.

STEP 2 = > What relevant data provided in this problem are necessary in order to answer the question?
Diagram 1 summarizes the information given in the problem.

STEP 3 = > Use the relevant data to solve the question.
The hypotenuse of the larger triangle shows the sight-line from point B to the tower top. The final elevation of the light on top of the tower must be the length of x plus 495 and the height of the tower is just that elevation minus the elevation of the ground where the tower sits.

The difference in height between point B and the hilltop is 42 m. Therefore, 42/100 = x/150 and the x in the diagram is 63 m above point B. This would put the top of the tower at an elevation of 63 + 495, or 558 m.
The base of the tower is on a contour line at 520 m, so the tower height must be 558 − 520 = 38m.

248   Answer D

STEP 1 = > What do you need to determine to solve the problem?
What ground distance will give a grade of 5%?

STEP 2 = > What relevant data provided in this problem are necessary in order to answer the question?
The elevations at point B and the hilltop.

STEP 3 = > Use the relevant data to solve the question.
The difference in elevations between these two points is 43 m. To get a 5% grade, 43/x = 0.05. Solving gives a minimum ground distance of 43/0.05 = 860 m.

249   Answer D

STEP 1 = > What do you need to determine to solve the problem?
The amount of memory left when the reserved memory is subtracted.

STEP 2 = > What relevant data provided in this problem are necessary in order to answer the question?
The total memory is given and the addresses for the reserved memory are given. Also, the amount of memory for each address is given as one word = two bytes.

STEP 3 = > Use the relevant data to solve the question.
The total number of memory addresses is hFFFF, which is d(256 x 256). The reserved memory is from hFF00 to hFFFF, or FF, which equals d(16 x 16) =256. Subtracting this from the total means that there are d(256 x 255) = 65280 addresses available to hold data. Since each address is one word, and each word is two bytes of data, 2 x 65280 = 130560 bytes available. This is closest to 130 Kb.

250   Answer B

STEP 1 = > What do you need to determine to solve the problem?
Determine what is changing with the sequence of put operations.

STEP 2 = > What relevant data provided in this problem are necessary in order to answer the question?
The values being moved and where they are being moved to and the distinction between an address and the value at that address.

STEP 3 = > Use the relevant data to solve the question.
The first put operation moves the value (unknown) at hFFFF to h1234. In essence, this is storing the current pointer value at memory location h1234. The next put operation moves whatever value (unknown) is at hEA34 into hFFFF. The last put operation moves the value at h1234 (still unknown, but this is the original value of hFFFF that was stored there in step one) into hFFFF.

The net result of these operations is to move the contents of the pointer to another location, then change the contents of the pointer to whatever is at hEA34 and finally to change the contents of the pointer back to what it was originally. The only thing that has changed is that h1234 has the original pointer value. Since we don't know what was in h1234 to start with, this may or may not be a different value.

251   Answer A

STEP 1 = > What do you need to determine to solve the problem?
What order will the data be in when the sequence is executed.

STEP 2 = > What relevant data provided in this problem are necessary in order to answer the question?
How FILO works, since the sequence is essentially one FILO operation followed by another.

STEP 3 = > Use the relevant data to solve the question.
If the following 4 data items are input and then moved and input somewhere else (both in FILO order) we have a,b,c,d (original order) → d,c,b,a (order in first memory location) → d,c,b,a (order sent to second memory location) → a,b,c,d (order in second memory location) → a,b,c,d (order of final output). This final ordering is FIFO.

252 Answer A

STEP 1 = > What do you need to determine to solve the problem?
What each step in the sequence does.

STEP 2 = > What relevant data provided in this problem are necessary in order to answer the question?
The pointer value is increased by one after each item is input. The value at hFFFF determines where the pointer points.

STEP 3 = > Use the relevant data to solve the question.
Step one moves the value at hAB25 (which we are told is h00A5) to hFFFF, this means the pointer is now pointing to h00A5.

The next step puts the data values given into memory, starting at h00A5. This also increases the pointer by the number of data items, so that it now points to h00AA.
The next step puts the value at h00A8 (which is one of the items just input) into hFFFF. The value at h00A8 (from the data list) is b111. This means the pointer is reset to point at b111, or, in hexadecimal, h0007.
The next step inputs the data again, starting with h0007 (which will contain b11) through h000B. After the input, the pointer will be pointing at h000C.
Since memory location h000B contains the last data item, b1000.

253 Answer D

STEP 1 = > What do you need to determine to solve the problem?
What does the graph imply about the nutrients shown?

STEP 2 = > What relevant data provided in this problem are necessary in order to answer the question?
The cumulative percentages of each nutrient and the cumulative percentage of dry weight and the time frame for each.

STEP 3 = > Use the relevant data to solve the question.
Since the cumulative percentage lines do not show actual weights for each nutrient (only the relative percentage uptake) no determination can be made about amounts. So (A) and (B) cannot be determined by this graph. Water absorption doesn't appear on the graph, so (C) isn't shown.
Because growth continues after all the potassium is taken up, potassium cannot be a major structural element for this plant, (D) is correct.

254 Answer D

STEP 1 => What do you need to determine to solve the problem?
Where and how would a line for the cumulative percentage of C, O and H appear on this graph?

STEP 2 => What relevant data provided in this problem are necessary in order to answer the question?
The relative percentages of C, O and H are given as well as the percentages of N, P and K.

STEP 3 => Use the relevant data to solve the question.
All lines must appear to the left of the Dry Weight line, since all elements are included in Dry Weight. However, since the sum of C, O and H is 96% of the Dry Weight, and the sum of the other nutrients shown is just 2.7%, on the resolution in this graph, a line for C, O and H would be indistinguishable from the line for dry weight already drawn.

255 Answer B

STEP 1 => What do you need to determine to solve the problem?
Determine how the available phosphate is replenished and subtract total phosphate need to find out how much additional is required.

STEP 2 => What relevant data provided in this problem are necessary in order to answer the question?
Conversion from Kg/hectacre to pounds per acre (one hectacre = 2.47 acres; one Kg = 2.2lb). The rate at which phosphate is replenished from non-fertilizer sources.

STEP 3 => Use the relevant data to solve the question.
1Kg/hectacre per week time 20 weeks = 20Kg/hectacre = 8Kg/acre = 17.6 lb/acre from soil reserves.
The total required is 25lb/acre; 25 − 17.6 = 7.4lb/acre.

256 Answer B

STEP 1 => What do you need to determine to solve the problem?
How much phosphate is being used per unit time as shown in figure one and when will the available soil phosphate run low?

STEP 2 = > What relevant data provided in this problem are necessary in order to answer the question?
Figure one shows how much P is being used over the growing period as a percentage of overall uptake. The total necessary is given and the amount from soil is given. By tracking weekly balances between plant needs and soil availability, we can find out where the soil runs low.

STEP 3 = > Use the relevant data to solve the question.
Since the overall usage is 25lb/acre each 10% increase for P in figure one is 2.5lb/acre. The soil provides 1Kg/hectacre = 0.9lb/acre per week. After 30 days, about 20%P has been used. This is about 5lb per acre. Over these 4 weeks, the maximum provided by the soil is 4 x .9 = 3.6lb/acre, so application of fertilizer would have to be before the 30 days. At 20 days, P usage is about 10% = 2.5lb/acre. Soil availability is 3 x .9 = 2.7lb/acre. Within the accuracy of figure one, this is the best estimate of the choices given.

257   Answer C

STEP 1 = > What do you need to determine to solve the problem?
The effect of increased pH on phosphate availability from soil sources.

STEP 2 = > What relevant data provided in this problem are necessary in order to answer the question?
We are told that ki and kb will increase with an increase in pH.

STEP 3 = > Use the relevant data to solve the question.
Raising the rate constants will increase the availability of soil phosphate which will change the amount of phosphate available. This will reduce overall fertilizer demand and allow a later application. The total amount and rate of use for P will not change, so the curve in figure one will remain the same.

258   Answer B

STEP 1 = > What do you need to determine to solve the problem?
The preference order B, C, A, D and an understanding of how a Condorcet ballot is marked.

STEP 2 = > What relevant data provided in this problem are necessary in order to answer the question?
The preference order and marking method: a 1 for a candidate preferred over any specific opponent and a zero otherwise.

STEP 3 = > Use the relevant data to solve the question.
Row one: Since A is only preferred over D and not preferred over any other opponent, the first row will be – 0 0 1. For the second row, B is preferred over all other choices and will have 1 – 1 1. This same procedure for the third and forth row yields (B) as the correct answer.

259   Answer **A**

STEP 1 = > What do you need to determine to solve the problem?
A pairwise comparison of candidates to determine an overall winner.

STEP 2 = > What relevant data provided in this problem are necessary in order to answer the question?
The summed ballot shown in diagram 2.

STEP 3 = > Use the relevant data to solve the question.
Since A loses against all opponents (first row), A is ranked last.
B wins against C (3:0) and D (2:1) and so B is first.
Finally, comparing C and D shows C beats D 2:1. The final ranking is then B, C, D, A.

260   Answer **D**

STEP 1 = > What do you need to determine to solve the problem?
Determine the number of votes in a pairwise manner given the percentages of voters who support a particular ranking.

STEP 2 = > What relevant data provided in this problem are necessary in order to answer the question?
The percentages and the preferred rankings.

STEP 3 = > Use the relevant data to solve the question.
Consider an election with 100 voters. By inspection, 45 will prefer A over all others. Similarly, 40 will prefer B, 10 C and 5 D. Pairwise, A loses to B because 45 prefer A over

Worked Solutions

B, but in total, 55 prefer B to A. B loses to C because only 45 prefer B over C and 55 prefer C over B.

C wins against B and D, but ties with A. The tie with A means that C doesn't win against all others. The election in this case doesn't have a clear Condorcet winner.

261 Answer C

STEP 1 = > What do you need to determine to solve the problem?
You need to fill out a summed ballot and total the rows to resolve any ties.

STEP 2 = > What relevant data provided in this problem are necessary in order to answer the question?
The percentages and the preferences listed in problem 3 allow a summed ballot to be generated.

		opponent			
		A	B	C	D	ROW TOTALS
candidate	A	—	45,0, 0,0 = 45	45,0, 0,5 = 50	45,0, 0,0 = 45	140
	B	0,40, 10,5 = 55	—	0,40, 0,5 = 45	45,40, 0,0 = 85	185
	C	0,40, 10,0 = 50	45,0, 10,0 = 55	—	45,40, 10,0 = 95	200
	D	0,40, 10,5 = 55	0,0, 10,5 = 15	0,0, 0,5 = 5	—	75

Diagram 3

STEP 3 = > Use the relevant data to solve the question.
Diagram 3 shows a ballot filled in with the rows totaled. It is generated for a 100 voter field so that the numbers equal the percentages given. For example, because 45 people prefer A over all other candidates, a 45 is entered in each box in the first row. The only

other voting group that prefers A over any other candidate is the last, which gives an additional 5 votes for A over C.

This is done for each candidate and then the totals are written down (in this case, each box's total is underlined). This completes the summed ballot for the information given. The rows are summed to settle any ties.
For clarity, data from each group is listed in order and separated by commas. As stated in the problem, row totals are only used to settle ties.

As before, C beats everyone but A, and now, the row totals (200 > 140) settle the tie. So the top ranked candidate is C. A loses to all the other candidates and is ranked last. Comparing B and D shows B beating D 85:15. The final ranking is C, B, D, A.

262 Answer C

STEP 1 = > What do you need to determine to solve the problem?
How does the ranking change for each voting group and how does this affect the election results?

STEP 2 = > What relevant data provided in this problem are necessary in order to answer the question?
Burying is defined and that definition is used to modify the data given in question 3.

STEP 3 = > Use the relevant data to solve the question.
The new ordering based on the definition of burying will be:

45% A, C, D, B
40% B, C, D, A (note that when B is the first choice, these voters do not bury B)
10% C, D, A, B
 5% D, A, C, B

The summed ballot changes based on these new numbers. B loses to all other candidates and will be ranked last. A and C still tie and the tie is resolved by a row total. C ranks first. A comparison between A and D shows that D beats A (55:45) and the final order is C, D, A, B.

Printed in Great Britain
by Amazon